The
ENGAGEMENT
DIET

Fit to Be Tied

The Complete HIS and HER Guide to
Getting in Shape for Your Big Day

BREAH HERZOG
and
CLINT HERZOG

INSPIRE™
ON PURPOSE
PRESS

Published by Inspire On Purpose™
909 Lake Carolyn Parkway, Suite 300
Irving, Texas 75039
Toll Free 888-403-2727
www.inspireonpurpose.com
The Platform Publisher™

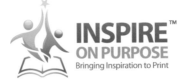

INSPIRE™
ON PURPOSE
Bringing Inspiration to Print

Printed in the United States of America
Library of Congress Control Number: 2011931544
ISBN 10: 0982562217
ISBN 13: 9780982562215

DEDICATION

We dedicate this book to all the couples who have traveled the road to good health together and to those who are on the verge of beginning this wonderfully challenging journey. Our deepest desire is that this book will transform your life and marriage through fitness. *The Engagement Diet i*s both a reflection of the struggles we have had in our relationship and homage to the progress we have made in developing a fit marriage. If we can play a small role in influencing others to have a healthy body and a healthy marriage for life, we will consider this book a great success!

ACKNOWLEDGEMENTS

We wish to thank our children, Parker and Hudson, who inspire us every day to be our best. Thanks to our family and the friends on our team, who passed the Mom Test, and loved us the whole way through. We wish to thank Jeff Crilley who first encouraged us to write this book, our trainer Sagi Kalev who coached us to a fitness level we never thought was possible, our photographer Robert Reiff who spent countless hours capturing images to inspire our readers, and our friend Robin Pou who played an integral role in the initial development of the manuscript. And finally, thanks to our publishers Michelle Morse and Terri Maxwell at Inspire On Purpose who helped us bring this book to print, but more importantly, who have truly embodied what it means to be part of the team. We love you all!

CONTENTS

APPENDIX

INTRODUCTION

Clint and I met each other in 2003 through mutual friends and were immediately head over heels. The funny thing is that we were both dating other people when we met. After six months, we eventually connected and the sparks were flying. Our first date was amazing! We both knew it was something special and we were in the right place to receive love from one another. We were engaged nine days later. Yes, I said nine days. We got engaged, planned a wedding and opened our business together all within four months. I know it sounds crazy, but at the time we just made it happen. We have now been married for seven years and have a four-year-old daughter named Parker and, more recently, a new baby boy named Hudson. What a fun ride!

After our daughter was born we were both in a fitness funk for a couple of years. This was really out of character for us—Clint and I had always been extremely athletic and in great shape. He was a former MMA fighter and I was a former Dallas Cowboys cheerleader. But when Parker came along, we were just going through life and putting ourselves, and our relationship, on the back burner. It seemed like we made every excuse in the book to not eat healthy or work out. With the new baby, we could also use guilt as a copout for not going to the gym. "Oh, we can't leave her," or "We can't take her to the kids' club." The truth is that we needed to be setting that healthy lifestyle example for our children.

Clint came home from work one day and told me he had stopped by the gym on the way home and signed up with a trainer. He shared that he was going to compete in a fitness competition in May, and he was really excited. At first, I was like, "What the hell?" I wanted to be angry and make it like he was getting to do whatever he wanted and I was just the mom at home with the kid that had no power to do what I wanted to do. The truth is, I had no idea what I wanted. I had lost myself in being a mom and had not been putting myself first. Clint told me he wanted me to do the competition with him if I was up for it. I said I would think about it.

I was overcome with fear and doubt. It's so funny how we can instantly talk ourselves out of something before we even think about it. Yet at that point, I knew I needed this for me. I knew we needed this as a couple to regain our passion for life. I knew if it was something I was running from for this long, then there was a huge breakthrough on the other side. I didn't know how it was going to look and Clint didn't either, but the thought of never putting it all out there was out of the question. I'd rather go all in and fail than play it safe and never know what might have been. We were not going to be paralyzed by fear. We both signed up for the competition—there was no backing out now.

We immediately began transforming our minds to prepare for the journey, changing the way we thought about food and fitness. We stuck with the program that our trainers developed for us, and our first fitness competition was five months later. I won first place in my division and Clint landed third in his. We were so pumped that we had committed to something together and stuck with it. Words cannot express the power this had on our marriage and our family. We continued competing on a national level and did extremely well. To look back and think about the day my husband came home and took a stand for us as a couple to be healthy and where it has now led us is amazing. I am so proud of him and respect him so much for taking that step.

Our relationship to food, fitness, and each other has transformed. We want everyone to have what we almost didn't have. We are writing this book to share our insights with our fans and readers, and inspire them to experience the same thrill of accomplishment that we discovered. Now that we are fulfilled, we can be the spouse, parent, and co-worker we have always wanted to be. We can give to others because we are full.

We hope that you discover the same joy and sense of empowerment from this program that we did when we first made the commitment to each other to get healthy together. We believe that doing The Engagement Diet as a couple can transform your relationship and let you experience a deeper level of closeness with one another as you prepare for your wedding day. May you be blessed with health, happiness and love throughout all the days of your marriage.

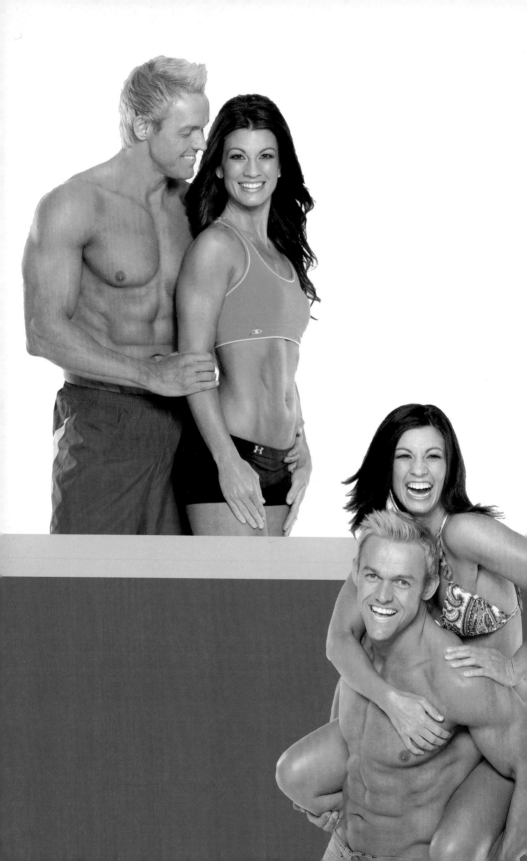

SECTION ONE

READY THE TEAM

A Message from Breah

Ladies,

Best wishes on your engagement and upcoming wedding! If you're like me, you probably feel like the weeks are flying by and there are simply too many things to get done in too little time before the big day. With so many matters demanding your attention, I want to congratulate you on pausing a moment to put yourself first, which is exactly what you did when you picked up this book and chose to start The Engagement Diet.

When I was in the middle of our wedding arrangements, I felt like there was not enough of "me" to go around. The wedding process is almost backwards. Naturally, it seems as if all things should be focused on the bride, yet, the process seems to require that the bride be there for everyone else—the mom, the in-laws, the florist, the church lady, the bridesmaids, and so on. Our schedules are tight, and when the end of the day comes, we discover that we have done little to focus on fitness.

As women, we have a tendency to put everyone else's needs first and settle for whatever scraps of time are left over for ourselves. But in doing so, we're really short-changing ourselves as well as the people we care about. I know that if I don't take care of myself, it is really hard for me to be there for others. And when it comes to planning a wedding, you will need an amazing amount of energy, stamina and patience to flat-out survive, let alone succeed.

That's why Clint and I wrote this book. We want you to succeed. When I look back on my own wedding day, I wish I had had a program like this. My wedding pictures are just okay. My friends and family are kind to think differently, but I know I wasn't in shape. There wasn't enough time to get it all done. So, the pictures are there—snapped once preserving that Breah for eternity. I will have those photos forever… sahweeet! My kids will see them. Their kids will see them. I cringe when our daughter wants to play wedding and asks to see them. Even though she is only four and thinks mommy is beautiful, I know they could have been better. I could have been better. That is one of my motivations for writing this book. I want you to have the wedding photos of your dreams.

More important than those beautiful pictures, though, I desire something else for you. What Clint and I now know—and what you will soon learn as you go through this program—is that as your commitment to fitness increases, so too does your commitment to each other. The transformation may look different for each couple, but getting fit together will make a lasting impact on your relationship. It did for ours. Through the pages of this book and the progress you will make with the program, you will discover this for yourself. I want to encourage you in that from the very beginning.

From the lessons I have learned, I want to help you find the time to focus on your fitness and to stick with it, especially during stressful times. You deserve to look and feel amazing on your big day, knowing you and your husband are fit to be tied.

Best,
Breah Herzog

A Message from Clint

Guys,

Hey, you did it. You're engaged. Congratulations!

Our engagement was a whirlwind. I popped the question after dating only nine days. Four months later we were married. It was crazy.

Once we were engaged, I began to realize that the groom is not really needed that much until the actual wedding day. That was a bit of a surprise. In my personal life, as in my career, I was calling most of the shots just up to the point that I asked Breah to marry me. I found the ring, I asked her dad, and I made the plan to pop the question. It was awesome—just as I planned it. Then, about an hour afterward, the wedding train revved its engines and didn't stop until we were practically comatose from exhaustion on the beach on our honeymoon. I wish I had been in better shape solely for the endurance…and for the honeymoon beach pics, too.

See, I was not that fit when we got married. On my wedding day I hated how I looked. I can see now that I dealt with the stress of the wedding planning by eating and drinking. There was no shortage of opportunities—the engagement party, wedding showers, bachelor parties, and so on. By the time the big day arrived, I could no longer do anything about the shape I was in. I want to spare you those feelings of regret. More importantly, I want to help you build an incredible foundation for your marriage by giving you new ways to communicate, encourage and support one another.

So now that your train has left the station, what are you doing to prepare for the big day? If you are reading this book, the person who gave it to you probably thought it was a good idea for you to get in shape for your walk down the aisle. Nice hint, huh? Well, I encourage you to take that hint and let it spark a fire to make a positive change in time for your wedding.

A Message from Clint

For me, marriage is great. Breah and I have a ton of fun. We love spending time together. Since our wedding, we have discovered that fitness, as a couple, is incredible. It adds so many elements to our relationship. I really had no idea.

Looking on the bright side, without that chubby hubby in the picture, we might not have had the incredible experience of getting fit together. And, I would never have been motivated to write this book. My goal is to coach you through your fitness journey from where you are today to the marriage altar. This book is your coach and guide.

I encourage you to do this program together. First, it wouldn't hurt to look your best for your big day. Really committing to this for yourself can be a wonderful wedding gift that you give your bride.

Second, she is super-psyched about the wedding. You want her to look her best. Supporting her in this fitness endeavor is a great way to say, "I love you"—and that's a great way to start the rest of your life with her.

Third, you get to do it as a couple. You'll both end up with fit bodies and ultimately a fit marriage. The two of you will look good, feel good and be proud of yourselves on one of the most important days of your life. You will be starting your marriage thinking, "Nothing can hold us back."

You Rock!
Clint Herzog

CHAPTER ONE

All for One:
It Begins with You

We wrote this book for a very specific reason. We love to help people see what is possible in their lives. Our identity as a couple is to strive to live a life we love. We know that when we take care of ourselves on all levels, we can truly be there for others. Of course, like everyone, each of us is still a work in progress. But we have discovered first-hand how fitness and food can affect your health and impact your relationships.

We did not have this program for our wedding day. We developed it after we were already married. Our motivation to get in shape came in the form of a fitness competition. Neither of us had ever competed in this type of contest. We did not think it was even possible. We talked to our trainer and decided almost as a joke that we would go for it. Not a super-confident way to start toward a goal, huh? Each of us had our reservations. What if one of us succeeded and the other did not? Finally, we said, "Let's commit to it and we will see." Every day we woke up and we had a choice to make: stay with the program or jump ship. Every day, we choose to stick with it. We also surrounded ourselves with people who supported our efforts and who believed that we could reach our goal. Their encouragement was invaluable.

To have the greatest chance for success in this program, you need support. Not just support from your future spouse, but from family and friends that you can count on to encourage you and hold you accountable. You need a team. We'll talk about who should be on your team in the next two chapters. First, we need to talk about you.

The Three Fundamentals

The program is twelve weeks long and is built on three fundamental elements: Fitness, Food and Relationship. The first two add stability to the third. When our food choices and our fitness are in line with our desired goals, our relationship takes on a new dynamic. We feel better about our own bodies, and we feel more passionate about our future spouse, because we have a shared bond of walking this journey together.

If you have corrected vision, you understand the difference a pair of glasses makes. Through your participation in The Engagement Diet, we are going to provide you with a new lens through which to view your relationship with food, fitness and each other. Your field of vision will be enhanced, and your outlook as a couple will subsequently improve. What better time to become closer than at the beginning of your marriage? The rewards will go on for a lifetime, and both of you are worth the effort.

We have created this very basic guide to take you step by step through three phases until you are both picture perfect for your wedding day. It will be a gift you give to yourselves, and each other, as a display of your commitment and love for one another. Don't worry— we are going to make it easy. After all, you are fit to be tied.

As with any activity that requires dedication and determination, you must first begin at the most basic place: you. From there you can begin to lay a foundation and work outward to build what it is you want. Start with the individual and build together as a team. We are here to coach and support you in every way possible so that you look and feel your best on the day you will cherish and celebrate for many years to come.

It Starts with You

The first part of recruiting your team starts at home. It starts with you. Take a good look in the mirror and pick you first. Recruit you. Imagine exactly what it is going to be like when you have completed this program and have experienced amazing results. Feel the pride of accomplishment. Own it. Victory is yours. Recruit yourself and hold on to that and hold on to what's possible for your life. Make a choice to put yourself first in this realm of fitness. Choose that you are going to do The Engagement Diet.

To be truly successful at this twelve-week program, you will need to plan. It's time to apply your wedding planning skills toward your grocery list and your fitness program! Be intentional and not reactive. Choose to make this program a top priority in your life in the same way that your other wedding plans are a priority. Before you worry about booking the band or choosing the flowers, take time to think about yourself and the goals you want to achieve.

Putting this program at the top of your "to do" list is vital to your success. Have you ever noticed that when you make something a lower priority, more often than not it doesn't get done? That's because by making it a low priority, you're essentially granting permission for it to get bumped from the list. You've determined that other things are more important. Working out is easy to put low on the list, but that's contrary to what you want to achieve. If you make your fitness a top priority, it will be less prone to getting bumped.

Maintaining Momentum

A lot of women—and even some men—will gravitate toward a crash diet to prepare for their wedding. Why? Because they are fast and they work. The bad news is, they can wreak havoc on your body. The crash-diet honeymoon is not pleasant. Landing on that beach tired, weak and starving is not the ideal romantic getaway. What's more, when you finish a crash diet, the pounds can pile back on just as quickly as they came off. Drastically cutting back on calories for the short term is a shock to your system, and your body wants to reset to "normal" as quickly as possible.

Twelve weeks may seem long for The Engagement Diet, but the timing is strategic. Your body has time to adjust to a new routine for your meals, and you lose weight gradually, which means it can stay off for good when you continue eating healthy. Plus, in twelve weeks, you can burn excess fat and develop lean muscle mass—which means you won't just be thinner, but also physically fit. You are transforming your body, and that doesn't happen overnight. When you're working the program, staying motivated throughout the twelve weeks is vital to your success.

Fortunately, motivation is built-in during this season of your life. You have a set day on which you are getting married. You know the exact time, the guests who will attend, the outfit you are going to wear and all the other details. In essence, all the elements of a well-defined goal are in place. Your goal is to be the best version of "you" that you can be as you walk down the aisle. Your motivation is evident by the fact that you are reading this book. Now, it's just a matter of choosing to stay motivated and stick with the program for the next ninety days.

To maintain your momentum, you can leave no room for doubt. As soon as you start to question whether the program will work, whether it's worth the effort, or whether you can make it all the way through, you leave the door open to look for an escape route. You begin giving yourself permission to quit.

We encourage you to focus on the excitement of what is possible. Push the doubt to the recesses of your mind. When you do The Engagement Diet with the person you love, it gives you the energy to support each other. Even doing it by yourself, you will discover that you have an inner strength that you never knew existed. So often, we look to the past and our life's history to define what is possible. "Both my parents are fat, so I'm destined to be overweight." "I've never been good at sports—I'm not going to do well with the exercise program." You probably have your own tapes playing in your head. We're here to tell you that the past is not the present. The past is not the future. Just because you have not done something in the past doesn't mean it cannot be done now.

If you replace the past with belief—belief that you can actually do this program—you can achieve great things. You can transform your body, and transform your relationship. All you have to do is follow the program. To maintain your momentum, focus on what is possible. Focus on what you are aiming for. Focus on your future together, as a fit and healthy couple, who continue to grow closer because you believe in each other and what you can achieve. When your momentum wanes, hold fast to the snapshot in your mind's eye of you and your beloved on your wedding day, looking better than you have ever looked, and feeling healthy and strong. This is your goal. You have the power to achieve it.

The Letter to Yourself

Along the journey of these twelve weeks, emotions can run the spectrum. At times you will find yourself excited and at other times you might just want to quit. This is normal and expected. You are doing something different. You are creating new routines in your eating and your fitness. This is helping define the type of relationship you have with your future spouse, since you have committed to do this together.

The excited emotions propel us forward. They leave us asking for more, striving to better our best. The I-wanna-quit emotions can be equally strong. Just know that they are typical, and that they pass just as some of the cravings you experience will pass, too. The usual pattern is that someone who wants to quit uses their team to help them rationalize quitting—why quitting is the right choice, the best choice and the only choice. If your team members are eager to help you throw in the towel, they shouldn't be on the team to begin with. That includes you. As the captain of your team, you hold the responsibility for generating excitement and momentum, and for pushing through the rough patches.

To accomplish your goals, it is good to be reminded of what you want to achieve, especially in the tough times. We recommend that you write down all the reasons why you want to do this program. Capture those thoughts now. Write yourself a letter. Be clear on why you are making this choice.

This letter to yourself is about possibility—your possibility. If you wipe clean the slate of assumptions of who you think you are, you can start from the fresh place of nothingness to create who you want to be—the new you. At times when you feel like you want to quit, you can pull out that letter. Read it and remind yourself of who you are, the commitment you made, and why you want this for yourself.

Share your letter with your partner. Ask them to remind you of your goals and your desire if they see you start to waver in your commitment. Their support will be invaluable.

Breah's Letter to Herself

I deserve this! I deserve to be healthy and happy. I have always wanted to push my body to the limit just to see what type of results I could achieve. I have so many emotions right now that I want to break through. I'm weary, doubtful, scared, overwhelmed and excited all in the same breath. I choose this diet and all of the great things that I believe will come out of it. Breah, don't let the negative little voice in your head tell you anything. You are not your past, but who you choose to be right now in this moment. You are a powerful woman and can do anything you set your mind to. You can do this and you can be a success at this. I am so grateful to be doing this diet with Clint. Together we will have each other to lean on and support. I know it will have an everlasting impact on our relationship and our lives. I can't wait. Let's get this party started. Bring it on.

Clint's Letter to Himself

You can do this. Twelve weeks to take your body to the next level is not a long time. When it gets tough, just remember how awesome the honeymoon is going to be, looking good and feeling great. This is not a chore but a gift to yourself. It is a chance to commit together for twelve weeks to a shared goal and love each other through it. It is going to be awesome and grueling at the same time, but ultimately awesome to reach the goal together and to see how you grow together as a result of the program. Most importantly, have fun. Play the game as if every last detail is extremely important while in the back of your mind, you know life is just not that serious. Channel that badass inside of you and *kick ass* for twelve weeks. It is worth it!

CHAPTER TWO

All for Two:
To Love, Honor and Cherish

The concept of commitment gets a lot of airtime during wedding season. It's the end result, right? In effect, you are committing all you are and all you have to someone else in "holy matrimony." Just by the fact that you are engaged, you understand what it means to commit to something or someone. In short, it's your word.

In the last chapter, we talked about making a commitment to yourself—making a pledge to do The Engagement Diet so you can look and feel your best on your wedding day. This chapter is all about the commitment you make to each other.

We believe true success requires support and motivation, and we have purposefully designed this program to be a couples' fitness program. A wedding is about two people coming together as one and promising to be accountable to each other throughout their marriage. By doing The Engagement Diet together, you have a chance to get a head start. You can be there for each other to support one another "for better or for worse"—trust us, you will see both!—and to motivate each other toward the goals each of you set in the program.

Do this together. Paint the picture for your future spouse of what is possible for the two of you. Acknowledge that you don't want to let each other down. Describe how you are going to hold each other's hand through the process. Rehearse this with each other so together you can recruit others to support both of you. In doing this, you are turning your future spouse into your XO. In military terms, XO is the Executive Officer, the second in command. Since you are striving to be first in command of your fitness, enrolling your XO is important to achieve your goals. And the acronym comes with a little kiss and hug (XO)—everyone needs that at the end of a hard workout.

Your word is your word. It's your bond. It's your integrity. Your word, like a muscle, can be strengthened with every commitment you make. Use this fitness program as strength training for your word in preparation for a lifelong commitment of marriage to the one you love.

You have an opportunity to commit to yourself and to your future spouse who you are (fit and healthy) and the support you offer. Here is a pledge you can make to each other.

Home Team Commitment

I commit to the twelve-week program with you.
I commit to myself to keep my word for the twelve weeks.
I commit to believing I can do it and renewing my commitment when I slip.
I commit to stand in love for your fitness goals by supporting you
    as XO in success, failure and in between.
I commit to listen to you for your possibility.
I commit to doing what I say I am going to do.
I commit to recruiting the "right" team.
I commit to taking the time to put me first.
I commit to being intentional in my daily and weekly planning for success.
I commit to asking for help.
I commit to communicating with my XO about all things related to the program.

Her Signature: _____ His Signature:_____

Today's Date: _____ Wedding Date: _____

If your commitment is your word, then that means something, especially within the bond of a relationship. Of course, committing to The Engagement Diet is not exactly the same as your marriage vows, but as you choose to do the program together, you are committing to one another. Any commitment to your spouse is important. In essence, you are inviting your partner to hold you to your word, and in the heat of battle when you want to quit, your beloved can remind you why you started this program. In an encouraging way they can help you remember down the road why you committed to this, what your goals are, and why they are important to both of you.

After the fitness competition, we continued working out and eating healthy. We got all kinds of questions about why we were continuing our healthy eating and fitness regime. People were confused. If the competition was over, why continue? For us, the answer was clear. Our confidence was soaring, because we had achieved our goal. We had more energy than ever before. We wanted to continue this throughout our lives. Getting fit for the contest was no longer something on each of our "to do" lists to be checked off, only to go back to our old ways. Our desire had changed. We had changed. We were transformed.

In the next chapter, we'll talk about building a team of supporters— people who "get" you and your goals—and how enlisting your army can help you achieve more than you could by yourself.

Breah's Insights

Doing the program as a couple, you may discover that how you like to be supported is not necessarily how your XO likes to be supported. We work hard to create a judgment-free zone—a safe place to fail and to just be there for one another. We have found that this, for us, is true support.

When, in love, one of us stands for the other who is heading down the slippery slope of poor choices, the effect is powerful. The one slipping may not get it at first, but we strive to be supportive in that, too. We focus on the fact that our choice is not necessarily their choice. This perspective allows you to demonstrate grace to your XO.

Clint's Insights

To truly support Breah, I needed to learn how she likes to receive support. I needed to identify the patterns of behavior that would allow me to engage with her in a supportive way. I discovered that we often give support in the way we like to receive support. I like to receive positive support, but this is not necessarily her support language.

Breah is not a fan of being told by me how to do her workout. I learned that if she did not do something in her workout, she did not want me to point out what she wasn't doing or what she should do. At first, I chose to just keep quiet. But I realized that my motive for staying silent was to avoid conflict and not to support my wife.

Eventually, I drummed up the courage to ask her how I could best be supportive while also holding her accountable. Now I have the language to approach her when I see she might be struggling, and to provide the type of feedback and encouragement that can help her move past hurdles.

CHAPTER 3
Three Cheers for the Team:
Enlist Your Army

When you commit to The Engagement Diet, your primary team is you and your future spouse. This is the training ground for your marriage. Two are becoming one. This is your forever team. Tackling your fitness is the perfect boot camp to prepare you for your life together.

But even in marriage, your world will not revolve solely around each other. You each have friends, family members and peers who play an important role in your lives. Why not let them in on the action?

Tell Others

Tell your family. Tell your friends. Invite your entire wedding party to join you in the program. Make it a whole big thing. Share your fitness goals with people that you believe are possible recruits for your support team. Life is a journey not meant to be travelled alone. We say, "You need a team." So, who's on your team?

For starters, think about your existing team—the people on your I'm-about-to-get-married team. Ask yourself whether they are good candidates for being on your getting-fit-for-your-wedding-day team, too. Some may be and some may not. You can go through this same exercise with your circle of friends and with your family. The goal is to recruit and enlist people that can truly support you. Planning your wedding is stressful enough—the details seem never-ending, and the days are fraught with distractions and filled with opportunities to make bad choices. Let down your defenses, and you can end up with a less-than-desired level of fitness on your big day. You need a team to watch your back—a trusted group of supporters who can help you stave off temptation and stay focused on your goal of looking and feeling your absolute best for your walk down the aisle.

In determining whom you should recruit for your team, we use a simple test: the Mom Test. Someone passes the Mom Test if they routinely get as excited about your goals as you do. They are genuinely excited about your successes without regard to themselves. They see your accomplishments for what they are from a passionate and loving perspective—just like your Mom does. Mom is the one who supports you no matter what. Your victories are hers. Your successes are hers. For you, who passes the Mom Test? Who are the Mom-worthy members of your team?

Choose Wisely

As you share the news about your choice to do The Engagement Diet, keep in mind that when others weigh in, sometimes their answer is more about them than you. Although you may believe they have your best interests at heart, their opinion about whether doing the program is a wise choice can be colored by their own struggles and personal history. Their input may inadvertently support that little voice of doubt in your head that is whispering, "You shouldn't do this. It'll take too much time. You'll miss all the fun of the wedding prep." As a result, you may just abandon the idea before you ever get started.

You might ask yourself how someone could not be on board with a fitness goal. All we can say is, it happens. We've seen it. You need to focus on what you know is right for *you* and surround yourself with people who support your choice to do something positive for your health, your self-image and your relationship. Chances are that when you chose to get married, you simply made a choice—you felt confident regardless of others' input. We encourage you to tap into that confidence and choose to commit to The Engagement Diet. Recruit the team that will cheer you on and help hold you accountable. Their encouragement and support can truly be life-changing.

We never could have made it to the fitness competition without the backing of our support team, and on the day of the competition, everyone we invited showed up—eighty members of our friends and family! They were there for us. We were overwhelmed to see how our decision to improve our physical strength and stamina made such an impact on others that they travelled all the way to Las Vegas to show their support. We were transformed, and their support further confirmed our commitment to who we now were. This was our "wedding day."

By completing The Engagement Diet in preparation for your wedding, you can demonstrate in a tangible way the strength of your commitment to your spouse, your team, and most importantly, to yourself. As loved ones give their blessing to you and your partner for becoming one, you will have already experienced an incredible journey together. You will already be "one," because you set a goal as a couple and stuck with it, supporting and encouraging one another along the way. As you say your wedding vows, you will look better, you will feel better physically, and you will feel closer to your new spouse than you ever imagined. Your team will be there to celebrate your success, just as ours was for us.

Rally the Troops

Our experience has shown that, unlike almost any other time, people are lined up to help during wedding planning season. They want a job. We say, "Let them in." Assign tasks to people on your support team. They'll derive great joy in knowing they helped in some way. Let them help while you go to the gym and eat right.

You may think that if you want something done right, you have to do it yourself. That's simply not true. Your friends, family and loved ones share a wealth of talent, and they are vested in your success.

Your army of recruits can help you if you let them. Delegation is key. You can't outsource your weight loss, and you need to reclaim some time to work out. So, ask yourself what you can outsource. What can you delegate?

Your army is not just there to bust you when you fail—although if you have the right recruits, sometimes it might seem this way. They will hold you accountable to the commitment you made and deliver "tough love" when needed. But your team is good for so much more. If they are for you then they will want to see you succeed. Part of your success should be to carve out the time you need to work out, so don't be afraid to ask for their help with the wedding logistics to help you free up time for the gym.

Once you are committed, you're "in." Once you recruit your team, you have committed to the program. Your commitment is your word. Your word is your bond. Once committed, you are set for success. We believe the true measure of a successful commitment is focus. When we focus, we succeed.

In the next section, we'll outline the tools for success when it comes to making smart food choices. We have created an easy meal planning system that will help guide your choices and keep you on track toward your goal for the next twelve weeks. The best part? You get a fun meal every once in a while. So get ready, because we're about to start an incredible journey.

Clint's Insights

When I first started this program with Breah, I experienced a rollercoaster of emotions about the changes it required. Digging deeper with the workout and food issues, I realized that I was hesitant to follow the program because I wanted to maintain control. I was fooling myself—I was not really in control to begin with. I was letting idleness and bad eating habits control me, and as a result, I was less than fit and healthy. When I gave up control to the program, I was set free. The results of sticking to my commitment are much better than the short-term gratification of sitting in front of the TV eating chips and cookies.

Breah's Insights

I know you have a lot of things on your mind with wedding planning. And now, you have committed to The Engagement Diet. You will experience times when you think you cannot do it—that you cannot see it through. I have been there. I totally get where you are. Give this to yourself. Give yourself this gift. You deserve it—the body you want, the wedding pictures you want, and the relationship you want. Give yourself permission to be selfish and do this for you. Your wedding day is about you and your fiancé. In this time, in the right way, put yourself first. If you don't take care of yourself, you will not be all you want to be for others in your life. Fill your cup.

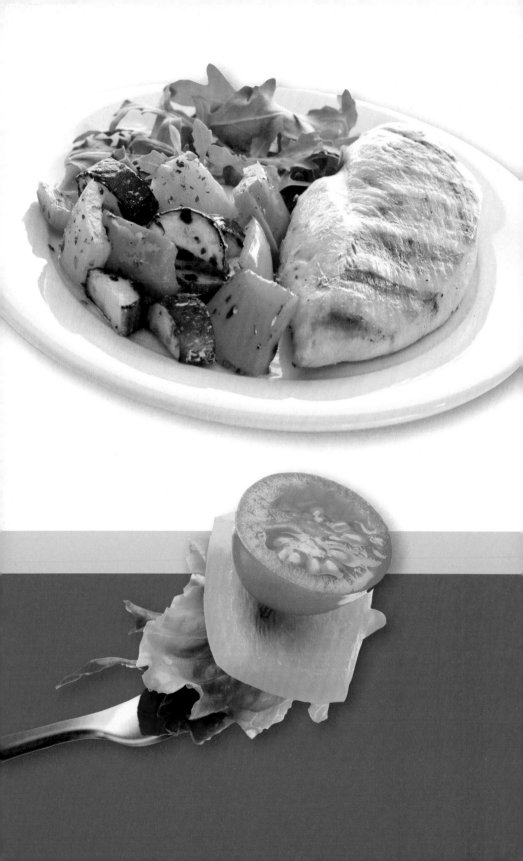

SECTION TWO

SET THE TABLE

CHAPTER 4
Quick Pick™ Meals:
Forget Counting Calories

Despite what it says on the cover, this is not a diet. Diets come and go. No weekly fad delivers lasting results. There is no magic pill. Trust us on this.

The Engagement Diet takes a holistic approach to getting in shape, which starts with learning to make smarter choices about what to eat while still really enjoying the food you love.

So often, we don't pay attention to what we're eating, or even why we're eating. Life is hectic—everyone is busy and we're perpetually multitasking. Finding time to focus on making good food choices can be a challenge. We eat mindlessly as we read emails, drive to an afternoon meeting, or watch television. We eat when we're bored or upset. We eat to celebrate special occasions. We eat whatever is quick and easy, or sometimes whatever is put in front of us. Our eating habits become completely unconscious. Rarely do these habits lead to a fit and healthy body.

Three Steps to Success

The Engagement Diet teaches you how to reprogram the way you think about food. It teaches you to be mindful, and to make conscious

Food

choices about what you are eating and when you should eat. When we first started on the journey to personal fitness, we turned to the experts. Nutritionists are experts in food. They have a ton of knowledge. As a result of the time we spent learning from nutrition specialists, we now know that if you want the best fitness results possible, dialing in the diet is key.

We took what we learned and broke it down so we could understand for ourselves and find a way to make it simple—simple enough to fit into our busy lives. Since our diet has a high impact on the progress of our fitness, we wanted a food program that would set us up to succeed. In short, we wanted to formulate an easy way to get on track and stay on track with our nutrition. Through years of working with trainers and learning to eat well, we have designed a food program that is as easy as 1, 2, 3.

Thus was born the Quick Pick™ Plan and our three categories of meal types:

> Number 1 – Fuel Meals
> Number 2 – Fair Meals
> Number 3 – Fun Meals

The food plan is laid out in such a way that you can incorporate it directly into your new fitness routine. Over the course of the program you will learn to discern which meals are which. The fundamentals are simple: eat small meals, make good choices and eat often.

Number 1 Meals

Number 1 meals are the best choice. They represent fuel for your body—fuel it will need to maximize the effort you are applying to your workouts. Number 1 meals pave the road to true body transformation, especially in the relatively short time frame of twelve weeks. They are comprised of lean protein, complex carbohydrates and leafy green vegetables. We love good food that is tasty. We have some suggestions we think you will enjoy to make your Number 1 meals something you look forward to.

Number 2 Meals

What we call Number 2 meals are those meals that most people think are healthy. If they were asked to rate them according to our scale, they might score them a Number 1 meal. But Number 2 meals are characteristically just fair from a nutrition perspective. They are not bad choices, but they are not the healthiest meal either. If you are working hard in the gym, help yourself out by making the best possible food choices at least for the next twelve weeks.

The best part about Number 2 meals is that you can always find them, even on the road. For example, if you are out at your favorite Mexican restaurant, you can eat a Number 2 meal. You just have to make conscientious choices. But once you pile on a load of sour cream and add a tortilla to your grilled chicken fajitas, you just went from a Number 2 to a Number 3 meal.

Number 3 Meals

You might be shocked to know that unlike the (now defunct) U.S. Government's Food Pyramid™, our chart calls for a fun meal or two every now and then. That's right, you get a break. We know you will need a break, because we needed a break. For us, it is just a reality, especially during such a hectic time as planning your wedding. Honestly, who can resist a really good cheeseburger or their favorite pizza? Not us. So, as a couple, we have chosen to no longer participate in any restrictive fad diet. We mentally need the reward to keep going strong, so we implemented the fun meal. It also gives you the psychological motivation to keep going with the program and spikes your metabolism so your body uses the fuel you put in more efficiently.

Number 3 meals are all about grace. They give you room to indulge. We want you to enjoy that burger or pizza and not feel guilty about it. Face it, when you are planning a wedding and attending all the festivities, you need to have a few fun meals planned here and there. If you have a cake tasting next week, then be sure your diet reflects the number of 1 and 2 meals you need to get that cake tasting as a

31

3. Remember, planning is key. Account for the fun meal and move on. You deserve it. Choose it. Plan it. Own it. The fun meal is a reward—a mini vacation from the program for one meal. Treating yourself once in a while is fine, as long as you are intentional with your choices.

Our goal is to help you develop a new relationship to food. When you start to think about the fun meal as a special treat and become more mindful of your eating habits, you become more confident and vested in the program. This enhances your motivation to see it through. Motivation and support—the keys to success!

Good Choices Rule the Day

The three meal categories work together over the course of the twelve weeks. We have put together a shopping list for each meal type in the next chapter. At first, your week's food plan will include more Number 2 and Number 3 meals, and then they will slowly taper off throughout the program. This helps in lessening the food shock to your system. As you progress week to week, you will add more Number 1 meals to your weekly food plan at the same time you lessen the number of Number 3 meals. You'll focus more on fuel for the new muscle tone you develop and move further away from old habits. We have found that as people get more nutritionally fit they want more Number 1 meals and experience a loss of the cravings for their Number 3 meals. As you transform your body, it starts telling you that you don't want the Number 3 meal. You start becoming more aware of what your body needs and you desire to fill that need.

More is Better

One of the best parts of the Quick Pick™ Meal Plan is that you actually get to eat more often. In fact, you will be eating five to six small meals a day, instead of two or three large meals. This way, you continue to add fuel to the furnace that is your metabolism. Taking in too much food at one time chokes the fire and slows your biological engine. You can also experience erratic spikes and drops in your blood sugar. (Ever had that experience of practically falling asleep at your desk about an hour after a heavy lunch?) By spacing out your meals and having smaller quantities each time, you can avoid the rollercoaster of highs and lows, stave off hunger pangs, and rev your metabolism to its maximum effectiveness.

The meal plan focuses on fresh foods—everything you would find in the outside aisles at the grocery store, like fresh fruits and vegetables— and avoids processed and pre-packaged foods. (Anything that can stay on the shelf for an extended period will also stay in your body for an extended period. We want to burn the calories we're taking in, not have them stick!) We will also focus on complex carbohydrates, like brown rice and sweet potatoes, which take longer to break down than simple carbohydrates, like breads, white rice and sweets. Your ideal meal will be a hand-size portion of lean protein (think chicken or fish), a fist full of complex carbohydrates (think broccoli or sweet potato), and a thumb-size portion of fat (like avocado, nuts, olives, or almond butter), which helps to lubricate the digestion. If you're the cook in the household, we recommend that you use a non-stick spray, instead of oil or butter, to save the fat grams. You'll also be drinking lots of water—regular soda is off the list, because you don't want to drink your calories and regular sodas are loaded with sugar—and you'll enjoy protein shakes as a snack to keep you feeling full and energized.

What to Expect

We'll go into more detail about how to plan your meals in the next chapter. We'll also share some tips on how to change your thinking about food and avoid common traps. For starters, though, here's a summary of what you can expect from the Quick Pick™ Meal Plan over the next twelve weeks.

Phase I (Weeks 1 to 4)

You will learn which foods fall into each meal category; i.e., Number 1 (fuel), Number 2 (fair) and Number 3 (fun) meals. You will phase into the program and become aware of what you are eating. You will begin to plan your food and fit it into your life. You'll adjust to the idea of eating five to six times each day.

Food

Phase II (Weeks 5 to 8)

At this point, you start to get it. You can begin to play with your food, figuratively. You will naturally gravitate to purer Number 1 meals and fewer Number 3 meals. As your body begins to transform, your food choices will become easier. Your results will create a drive in you to make better food choices. You will start to crave healthier foods rather than the unhealthy choices.

Phase III (Weeks 9 to 12)

You are dancing on the borderline of a lifestyle change. You will feel the breaking of any addictions to food you might have had. A new relationship to food is on the horizon. You are aware of how different food choices make you feel. You are committed to success.

Clint's Insights

I have been through my fair share of trainers. I kept changing trainers because I wasn't getting the results I wanted. These were good trainers, too. The reason my body wasn't transforming in the way that I desired, it turned out, was because I wasn't doing what they told me to when it came to food. Food is it. It is the road to success. Your workouts are hard enough without also bearing the burden of over-compensating for poor food choices. For results in twelve weeks, food is 80% of the equation.

Breah's Insights

Set a goal to self-regulate on food. Become aware of how different foods make your body feel. For example, determine which foods you cannot digest or cause you to bloat. Your body has chemical reactions to different foods. Before the two of us really started paying attention to this we had no idea. We would basically throw a bunch of stuff in the tank and expect the engine of our body to perform. Looking back on it, we do not really remember feeling bad. The problem was that we felt chronically bad. That was our baseline—feeling bad was our "good," because we didn't know that we could feel any different. As we changed our eating habits, we began to understand that we did not have the first clue as to what healthy felt like. After completing the program we never knew feeling great could feel this great. Our entire frame of reference changed. Yours will, too, and you'll love it.

CHAPTER 5
A New Routine:
Small Changes, Big Results

Developing a new relationship to food requires an investment of time up front to ensure good food choices. Set yourself up to succeed by planning your meals for the week in advance, including your fun meals. By planning your food choices in advance, you are more likely to stick with the program and to achieve the long-term results you desire.

As you begin to think about building your meals according to the Quick Pick™ Meal Plan , you need to know which foods fall into which categories. We have included a food appendix in the back of the book with a list of food options and the category—1, 2 or 3—into which each falls. Take a look at the list and find your favorite foods and their corresponding categories.

Now, look at the calendar and determine what you will eat for each meal every day for the next week. You can find a Quick Pick™ Meal Planner template in the appendix. Plan every meal. This may seem a bit hardcore, but we've found that this level of detail gives couples more confidence as they adopt a new routine. It gives them an opportunity to say no to poor choices when they arise. They are prepared. You can be prepared, too. According to which phase of the program you are in, take these steps to complete your Weekly Quick Pick™ Meal Planner and incorporate the right amount of Number 1, 2 and 3 meals into your weekly diet.

Step 1: Look at the calendar and determine when you are going to indulge in your Number 3 meals. Remember to plan around events like wine parties and cake tastings. Schedule your fun meals first, according to the phase of the program you are in that week.

Step 2: Fill in all your Number 1s first. Remember, these meals are the ones you can really control. Check your work calendar to see when you have client lunches and other events that might put you at risk of not achieving a Number 1.

Step 3: Fill in the rest of the meals with Number 2s. Remember, these are fair choices. You can still make basically healthy choices wherever you are.

The Choice is Yours

At its core, this program is designed to introduce you to a new kind of relationship with food. Regular exercise is part of the plan, but changing the way you think about eating and the choices you make are essential to achieving your goal of looking and feeling fantastic on your wedding day. When you think about Quick Pick™ meals, we want you to keep two things in mind: *food choice* and *food portions*. If you choose correctly and choose the right amount, then victory is yours.

Regarding the food choices, your focus will be on proteins and carbohydrates when putting meals together on the Quick Pick™ plan. The proteins should be lean meats, such as fish, turkey or chicken. Fatty proteins, like hamburger meat and pork, are not good choices. Likewise, you want to choose complex carbohydrates, such as brown rice and green veggies. Simple carbs, like chips and white bread, can actually throw your metabolism out of whack. Finally, your fat intake should come from things like olives, nuts, beans or avocados. (Fat contains more calories per gram, so it takes much less fat to meet your daily needs.) Avoid fat from fried foods, fatty meats, and butter.

Fueling Your Body

You might find it odd that you eat more frequently while following The Engagement Diet. Science tells us that eating small meals five to six times per day actually keeps your metabolic fire burning and helps sculpt lean muscle and shed fat. The key is to eat smaller portions several times a day, rather than scarfing down a huge meal that puts you in a food coma. Meals will be a different size for different individuals, but the simplest measuring tool to use is your hand. Any given meal should include a portion of protein no larger than the palm of your hand, a portion of carbohydrates no larger than the size of your fist, and a portion of fat no larger than the size of your thumb. At each meal, your calories should be divided proportionately between 40% protein, 30% carbohydrates and 30% fat. This will provide enough protein for lean muscle, the right complex carbohydrates for energy, and healthy fat for digestion. Any of these out of whack can spell disaster.

Shopping Smarter

Because you are busy planning your wedding while continuing to do the other things in your life (you know, go to work, spend time with friends, and so on) we wanted to make this program super-simple and set you up to choose your food well. Planning a wedding puts enough obstacles in your path to keep you from getting fit. We didn't want to add "difficult" to that list. So, in keeping with the goal of being easy and simple, we have listed meal suggestions and created a grocery list for each category of meal (Number 1, Number 2 or Number 3). This list includes all the food in the Quick Pick™ Meal Plan organized into categories you would find at the grocery store. We encourage you to use these lists for the next few weeks to continue your week-to-week planning.

Number 1 Meals Grocery List

PROTEIN

Cod	Tilapia
Egg whites	Tuna
Orange roughy	Turkey
Salmon	White chicken
Sea bass	

COMPLEX CARBS

Arugula	Cream of rice
Asparagus	Cucumbers
Black beans	Green beans
Broccoli	Green peas
Brown rice	Greens (salad)
Brussels sprouts	Oatmeal
Carrots	Spinach
Cauliflower	Sweet potato
Celery	Zucchini

SNACKS

1 tbsp almond butter	Green apples
Blackberries	Greens (salad)
Blueberries	Oatmeal
Broccoli	Raspberries
Carrots	Raw almonds
Celery	Small piece of protein
Cranberries (unsweetened)	Spinach
Cucumber	Sweet potato
Grapefruit	Flavored high-grade
Greek yogurt (add protein	protein powder shake
powder and sugar substitute)	Zucchini

SPICE IT UP

Ketchup
Mustard
Peppers
Pickles
Salsa
Salt
Pepper

Use: Cooking spray instead of oil or butter

Add: Tomatoes, mushrooms, onions, spinach, etc. to egg whites or ground turkey

DRINKS

Coffee
Tea (hot or cold)
Diet soda
Light sugar-free drink
Water or sparkling water

Example Number 1 Meals

Remember, your ideal meal will be a hand-size portion of lean protein (think chicken or fish), a fist full of complex carbohydrates (think broccoli or sweet potato), and a thumb-size portion of fat (like avocado, nuts, olives, or almond butter), which helps to lubricate the digestion.

This method makes it very easy to measure your food without having to whip out of your back pocket a scale or measuring cups and spoons. We specified cups and ounces in the examples below, but that is just for a frame of reference.

Food

Food

BREAKFAST

1/2 cup to one cup of cooked oats with handful of blueberries
1 piece of turkey bacon
Coffee, black or with artificial sweetener

Egg white omelet with tomatoes, onions, and spinach
1/2 cup to one cup cooked oats, plain or with flax seed
Iced tea, plain or with artificial sweetener

2 scrambled egg whites
2 pieces of turkey sausage
1/2 cup to one cup of cream of rice with handful of raspberries
Hot tea, plain or with artificial sweetener

LUNCH

Turkey breast (6-8 oz) with one cup of brown rice
Light sugar-free drink or water

Grilled chicken breast (6-8 oz)
Cup of mashed sweet potatoes
Sparkling water

Seared tuna salad w/ clear nonfat dressing
Cup of brussels sprouts
Iced tea, plain or with artificial sweetener

DINNER

Grilled chicken (6-8 oz) salad with clear nonfat dressing
Diet soda

Grilled chicken breast (6-8 oz)
Cup of cauliflower
Iced tea, plain or with artificial sweetener

Grilled tilapia (6-8 oz)
Cup of broccoli
Water

SNACKS:

Green apple with1 tbsp of almond butter
Grapefruit with artificial sweetener
Greek yogurt with a scoop of protein powder and artificial sweetener

We have created a Quick Pick™ Meal Plan broken down in phases to help you track the amount of Number 1, 2 and 3 meals you should include in your diet each week in order to achieve optimum results. As a convenient reference, you can also find the Quick Pick™ Meal Plan and Food List in the Appendix along with lots of tips about food.

Quick Pick™ Meal Plan by Numbers

Weeks	#1 Meals	#2 Meals	#3 Meals	Snacks
1 to 4 Phase One	14/week	5/week	2/week	14/week (2/day)
5 to 8 Phase Two	16/week	4/week	1/week	14/week (2/day)
9 to 12 Phase Three	18/week	2/week	1/week	14/week (2/day)

Remember: Your body is like a furnace, and your metabolism burns the fuel that you put inside. You can burn energy more effectively when you feed the fire throughout the day with several smaller meals and snacks, rather than eating a huge meal (a big log) that will put out the fire. That feeling of being in a food coma after you eat a huge meal is evidence of the way it shuts down your system. Small meals keep that metabolism up and burning those calories.

If you want to really dial it in, then just drop your Number 3 meals during the last two weeks to really turn up the heat.

For more tips, tools and information about The Engagement Diet, please visit our website at www.theengagementdiet.com.

Number 2 Meals Grocery List

PROTEIN

Lean red meat (filet mignon, New York strip)
Deli meat
Pork chop

CARBS

Pinto beans
Wheat pasta
White potatoes (plain)
White rice
Whole grain bread

Adding a small portion of these items will turn your Number 1 meal into a Number 2 meal:

Bananas	Pears
Cashews	Pecans
Grapes	Pistachios
Oranges	Plums
Peaches	Walnuts
Peanuts	1 tbsp. peanut butter

Example Number 2 Meals

BREAKFAST

Egg white sandwich on wheat bread
Cup of fruit
Coffee, black or with artificial sweetener

2 eggs over easy
1 piece turkey sausage
Wheat toast
Water

LUNCH

Turkey sandwich on wheat with mustard and veggies (no cheese)
Iced tea, plain or with artificial sweetener

Grilled chicken fajitas with thumb-sized portion of guacamole (no tortillas)
Side salad with clear nonfat dressing
Diet soda

DINNER

Turkey with whole-wheat spaghetti pasta in light marinara sauce
Iced tea, plain or with artificial sweetener

6-8 oz filet of lean red meat
Baked potato
Iced tea, plain or with artificial sweetener

SNACKS

There are no Number 2 snacks. Refer to your Number 1 snack list for all your daily snacks.

Remember: NOT ALL CARBS ARE CREATED EQUAL! Simple carbohydrates are broken down quickly and easily converted to fat. Examples of simple carbs include tortillas, chips and breads. Complex carbohydrates are broken down more slowly and allow the body to burn them off, minimizing their conversion to fat. Examples of complex carbs include broccoli, green beans, and leafy green vegetables.

Example Number 3 Meals

We are just going to give you a few ideas here. For a Number 3 meal you can enjoy one or two slices of pizza and a soda, a double hamburger with a half side of fries, two sour cream enchiladas and a side of rice and beans, or short stack of pancakes with powdered sugar and syrup and small glass of chocolate milk. You get the idea. Just don't go overboard, and always watch your portions.

Number 3 Meals Grocery List

You didn't really think we were going to give you a grocery list for the things you ideally should avoid, did you? Odds are, many of the items you shop for regularly qualify as a Number 3 type of food, including white bread, chips and thick salad dressings. You don't need to cut these out of the equation completely—that's what the fun meals are for—but remember, while you're doing The Engagement Diet, you are focused on the goal of eating healthy and getting fit. We recommend that you not keep many Number 3 foods in the house, so you won't be tempted in a moment of weakness!

So how do all these meals come together during the program? Here is the schedule for you to follow as you plan your meals during each phase of The Engagement Diet.

Two Heads are Better than One

When you're both on board with the program, developing new habits and routines together can be fun. After all, you are laying the foundation for your new life together—a life built on mutual support and encouragement, in which you both continually strive to be your best. Learning to plan your meals is a vital part of the new routine that will set you up for success. Some couples take planning to an art form. Here are a few tips from friends who have done the program, too.

- Shop for groceries at the beginning of the week.
- Cook your proteins for the week in advance.
- Pre-pack your meals in to-go containers together with plastic silverware.
- Pack snacks in plastic baggies to carry in your briefcase, purse or backpack
- Stock your snacks in places you will be throughout the week, including your home, office, and car.

Many couples have found that Sunday is the best day to go grocery shopping, because they often have more time on that day than during the rest of the week. Why not make it a date and go grocery shopping with your future spouse? This will set each of you up for the week with all the things you need to make good food choices and stay with the program.

Now it's time to take planning to a new level by determining the best places to eat out, how to avoid food traps, and what to do when you've exceeded your fun meals for the week. Don't worry, we've got your back!

Food

Clint's Insights

Growing up, my older brother was a pretty muscular guy. I basically lived the first 32 years of my life believing that he was the muscle guy and I wasn't ever going to be built like him. To live in that world, I made up stories. For example, my roommate in dental school was lean. I made up a story that he had a great metabolism. I believed it. It was make-believe. He would eat dessert with me, but when he was not with me he ate healthy. I just didn't see it. What I could not see allowed the story to survive.

Another story I told myself is that I couldn't lean out. That's when you reduce your body fat so you have a more sculpted look, and you get those six-pack abs everyone admires. I could always add muscle but I never could lean out. The truth was I didn't want to do the work. I didn't want to do cardio or eat right.

I never stuck to what I was supposed to in order to find out what I could achieve. I never followed the program long enough to see what the true outcome could be. As a result, I felt stuck. So, I said, "Screw it. Why even do it?"

It wasn't until I ultimately made a commitment to myself—and to Breah—to be "all in" that I finally saw the results I never thought were possible. I committed to following the instructions from my trainer and nutritionist and sticking with the program until I reached my goal, no matter what. The result? I looked better and felt better than I had my entire life. I got lean. I got ripped. I achieved my goal and felt like a champion. If I can do it, you can do it, too.

Breah's Insights

Chicken fried everything. That was the menu of choice at our house when I was growing up. Sloppy Joes were my leafy greens. My dad was the cook, so we ate whatever was easy to fix and it was never healthy.

Fast forward to my adult life. I left home and went to college. In my third year, the weight started to stick. It finally had caught up with me. My metabolism had slowed down. My lazy calorie-burning machine could not keep up with the intake.

I was blessed to have an aunt who stepped in and invited me to the gym. I started working out regularly and then changing my eating habits. I opted for healthier foods. I was cooking for myself, and I was making smarter choices. I changed my relationship to food and fitness. It felt incredible.

Your family's history and habits don't have to dictate what you see in the mirror. It's time for a fresh start. You deserve to look and feel your very best, especially on your wedding day. I am here to give you the know-how and the tools to achieve that goal. We'll make it happen.

CHAPTER 6
Time for Fun:
Indulge, but Be Honest

The Engagement Diet is designed to transform your body in twelve short weeks. When you work the program, you will see changes you never thought possible. Since we've been through the program, we understand that sticking to the guidelines can be challenging at times. That's why we created fun meals. We encourage you to take a walk on the wild side once in a while. The only caveat is that you plan when you will have a little fun. In other words, you should plan your Number 3 meals in advance. That way, you will know when you are done taking a break and can get back on track with your Number 1 and Number 2 meals.

Giving yourself the grace to indulge on occasion can help you stay motivated throughout all twelve weeks of the program. What's more, treating yourself to a piece of fried chicken once in a while can actually help you lose weight in the long run. It may seem counterintuitive, but when eaten sporadically and in conjunction with an otherwise nutritionally healthy food plan, fun meals can actually spike your metabolism!

Just how do you go about planning how to have some fun with your food choices? Here are a few tips.

Case Your Favorite Joints

A lot of our couples do not spend time cooking. If you and your future spouse fall into this group—or if you just want options for eating away from home that conform to the Quick Pick™ Meal Plan—you can study up on the menus for your favorite restaurants to determine which ones are the best choices while you're working the program.

Everyone has a treasured go-to breakfast joint, favorite lunch spot or fantastic mom-and-pop dinner restaurant. Take your newfound education about food to each of your regular places. Build a meal that fits your need—either a Number 1 or Number 2. Now, whenever you go there, you have a "safe" meal you can order. If you are a regular, you can even enlist the wait staff to help you by telling you how a certain food is prepared or healthy substitutions for menu items. You can recruit them to be on your team.

Eat, Drink and Be Wary

Temptation is everywhere. Stay on guard! Don't let common food traps trip you up and change your planned Number 1 meal into an unexpected Number 3 meal in the blink of an eye. Here are a few things to watch for:

- Tortilla chips at a Mexican restaurant
- Bread, rolls and breadsticks
- Mayo and BBQ sauce, both of which are high in sugar
- High-fat salad dressings, like ranch, blue cheese and Thousand Island
- Shredded cheese, sour cream, and other dairy-based toppings

If any of these things drop your meal to a Number 3, that's fine, right? But if it wasn't planned then you didn't even get to enjoy it as a Number 3 meal. And that other Number 3 meal later in the week might have to be bumped.

At this point, you might be asking yourself, "Does it really matter if I have an extra Number 3 meal? I mean, overall I am eating healthier than I did before." You do have a valid argument. It's not an issue of whether it "really matters," rather it's about the commitment you made. And one extra fun meal could lead to another. Suddenly, you look up and you're just not really doing the diet. You feel frustrated and ashamed, and rather than get back on the program, you decide it's easier to quit. The best way to prevent this from happening is to be mindful of everything that goes in your mouth—to plan your meals in advance and keep your guard up for unexpected traps. Remember, you're in control! Your goal is within reach; all it takes is persistence.

And Then Life Happens

Of course, we recognize that the best made plans still get messed up. Here's a funny story from our own experience. One night we were at our favorite Mexican food restaurant. We were eating clean. We had found the right food choices at our joint. We knew that we could eat clean or have a fun meal—we felt so empowered! That night we had chosen to eat a Number 1 meal.

Out of nowhere a new waiter brought us *queso*. We didn't order it. He said, "Oh, Monday nights are free *queso* night." We looked at each other and started cracking up...seriously? What are the odds? If it had been a fun meal night, they would have been out of freaking *queso*. Both of us started down the treacherous trail of temptation. *Hmm... what should we do? It's free for goodness' sakes.* Then we ordered fajitas for two, and guess what happened? Oh yes, you got it! With our double fajitas we got two free margaritas and *sopapillas* for dessert. You guys know the deal. Temptation arises at the right times to see if you are really going to keep your word. What's a couple to do? Is the world out to destroy our plans to get fit?

We ended up choosing not to eat the bad stuff even though it was free. Just because something is free doesn't mean it tastes better. Isn't it funny how our minds associate that free is better? It's like when you go to the movies and stay until the end, even though the film was really bad, because you paid for the ticket. In the end you "save" the money but waste the two hours.

Although this Mexican food night might have been a temptation before, we were in Week 10 of the program and we were committed. We sent it all back—the *queso*, the drinks and the dessert. Even though we had a fun meal to use, we just did not want to use it. When we left the restaurant we had broken through a barrier that would forever impact us in this program. We were saying no from a place of power. That is a place we want you to discover!

Inevitably, you will find yourself in a similar scenario, staring temptation in the face. Maybe everyone at the office is going to lunch. You want to be part of the bunch, but you planned your fun meals and this one wasn't on the calendar. Regardless, you go out. The group is going to an Italian restaurant. Stick with the program. Plan for the unexpected by knowing your go-to items for impromptu meals when you are out. The best part about almost every restaurant is that they have salad and grilled chicken. These are good choices. If everyone else is ordering fettuccini with Alfredo sauce, don't let yourself get caught up in the energy of the group. End the conversation in your head before it starts. Make the choice before you walk in the door. Don't even gaze over the menu. Order what you want.

As an added defense, leave a couple of Number 2 meals in reserve. Over-budget your Number 1 meals and under-budget your Number 2 meals. You never know what is going to pop up in your schedule, whether it's dinner with an important client, an impromptu party, or a friend who insists on taking you to lunch. Hold an extra Number 2 meal in your hip pocket to create the flexibility you need stick to the diet.

Clint's Insights

Food and fitness work hand-in-hand. If you already go to the gym regularly but aren't seeing the changes you desire, following the Quick Pick™ program will take you to the next level. By eating nutritious foods and eating smaller meals, several times a day, you rev-up your metabolism and switch out fat for muscle. The shape of your body will change.

Breah's Insights

Fitting into your skinny jeans isn't the only goal of The Engagement Diet. If you are skinny in the mirror but unhealthy inside, where does that leave you? We call this "skinny fat"—your body is slim, but you're not in shape, and you are putting the wrong kind of fuel into the engine. If you commit to the program, you will discover amazing physical results. Not only will you be toned and fit, but your skin will look better, your attitude will improve, and you'll have more energy to get through the day.

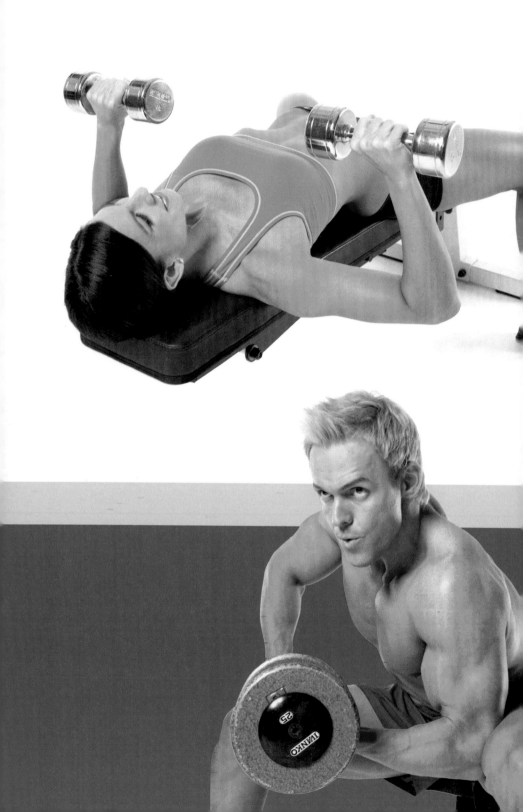

SECTION THREE

Go Build Some Muscle

CHAPTER 7

Fitness A:
Get a Plan!

Just as with the food portion of the program, we have designed the fitness portion to accommodate a busy schedule. To do this we believe you have to make it stupid easy. The Engagement Diet fitness regimen is designed to take you from where you are currently to getting your muscles back in shape. And it only takes five hours a week—just one hour per day, five days a week. Did you know that five hours is only 3% of your entire week? Imagine a 3% investment for a lifetime return. That's a pretty good deal, right?

Fitness ABCs

We also put together a fitness program that is sustainable long term. If it can be done long term, it can be done for twelve weeks. The program fits your everyday life.

The twelve-week duration was created by design. Over the course of the program, the workouts gradually become more intense, giving your body time to adapt. As you get stronger, we will crank the dial.

The workouts are designed to develop lean muscle mass to sculpt your body. The one-hour workout is comprised of two equal thirty-minute halves:

- thirty minutes of interval cardio – High Intensity Interval Training (HIIT)
- thirty minutes of weight training

This level of effort is more than sufficient to reach your goals as the program is designed to maximize efficiency in each of the thirty-minute segments—provided you stick with it. Consistency over the twelve weeks is the name of the game, both in your food choices and in your fitness. So, plan your workout schedule to accommodate your calendar. Our Fitness ABC Guide is conveniently located in the appendix. There you will find visual depictions of a variety of exercises along with specific details on what area of the body to train, when to train and for how long.

Get Your Clothes Out

Pull out your gym clothes. Pack your bag. You are ready to work out. Planning your time to exercise is just as important as planning your food. It might even be harder. For example, if you are not a morning person, but you realize that this is the only time in the day that you actually control your schedule, getting up early might be an adjustment. If you like to work out in the afternoon, how will you plan for the unexpected late meeting at the office? What about things that just pop up—the impromptu invitation to do something fun after work that precludes time to hit the gym? If you think about these types of scenarios in advance, you can be better prepared to deal with them when they come up.

Plan Your Fitness

Make your workout part of your weekly routine. Weekends are hectic and filled with parties and wedding planning. Ensure consistency to meet your goals by working out Monday through Friday. Many a couple have adopted this tactic and celebrated their week's accomplishment with a fun meal on Friday night.

The easiest method is to allot specific times to work out during the week. Put them on your calendar as appointments that you will not break. Think of this as your time. Pick the times and hold to it. Make the space for it. If you set your workout at the same time every day, you'll quickly develop a routine. It becomes rote—something you do habitually, just like brushing your teeth at night. You don't even think about it. You just do it.

Here are several other recommendations to help you incorporate your workouts into your daily life and stick with the program for the next 90 days.

- **Tell your team.** Let your office, family and friends know that you are unavailable during your workout. This single hour out of each day is for you and only you. Make the time as important as your commitment to it. Guard it, so you can be there for them and be at your best at those times when they need you.

- **Look forward to that time.** It's all about you—a gift you are giving yourself. It's not another thing to check off your daily list. It is quite the opposite, an oasis in your day. The time you give to yourself that expands the time you have for the rest of your day because you have taken care of you first.

- **Get comfortable at the gym.** If you have not yet joined a gym, you can often get the first session free, and a trainer will be happy to orient you as to the use of the various machines. Let them in on what you are doing. Enlist their support, regardless of whether you hire them to train you personally. They are there to help you. Use that resource. They will help you feel more confident entering the gym community and getting more comfortable with the surroundings.

- **Be intentional.** It is no accident that any of us are out of shape. The reverse is true, too. You are not going to accidentally get fit. Proactive intentionality is a good quality to have when you want to make a positive change.

- **Dress for success.** Look the part. Envision yourself in twelve weeks. Who do you see? Outfit that person with the clothes needed to be victorious. The goal is to feel good about going to the gym. Dress to accomplish that goal.

- **Buy some music.** Make a playlist that encourages you to new heights each and every day. Inspiration comes in many forms. If you like listening to music while you work out, you will be amazed at how just the right lyric to just the right song comes on at just the right time to push you to the next level.

- **Put your best foot forward.** Good shoes make all the difference. As it relates to clothing, splurge in this area. Go to your local athletic shoe store and tell them what you are doing. Have them size your feet and put you in the right brand shoe for your foot, your size, pronation and level of activity. You will enjoy having a shoe that supports you properly.

- **Get the gear you need.** If you are working out at home instead of at a gym, here are the things you will need to follow our twelve-week fitness plan:
  – Stackable dumbbells or resistance bands
  – Exercise ball
  – Medicine ball
  – Mat
  – Pull-up bar

What to Expect

Get ready to be transformed. When you stick with the Quick Pick™ Meal Plan in combination with The Engagement Diet fitness program, your body will begin to show results right away. You might not notice any changes in the first two weeks, but by weeks three and four, you will find your clothes are getting looser, you have more energy, and the workouts are getting easier to manage. The program is designed to gradually take your body step by step to a higher level of fitness. Here's a breakdown of how it looks.

Phase I – Stir It Up (Weeks 1 to 4)

Here is where you get your muscles ready, adjust your body to the program and really begin to stir things up. You'll be ramping into your new routine and getting comfortable with the exercises. Your muscles will be stirred up in order to help them reorganize. You'll be doing something that you might not have done in a while. You'll probably be really sore at first. You might even want to quit. Think of the soreness as your body communicating with you. It is saying that the process is working. Stick with it.

Phase II - Shape it Up (Weeks 5 to 8)

You are starting to shape up. The program is structured to tax muscles specifically for the goal of definition and tone. The Engagement Diet is designed to melt away the fat while building and maintaining lean muscle tone.

Phase III – Dial It In (Weeks 9 to 12)

You are really dialing it in now, shrink-wrapping it all for your ultimate goal. Your Big Day is in view. You naturally desire to be super-strict on the workout, getting rid of the last bit of excess fat. The difference in your strength is noticeable. The exercises are matched to your new strength.

Fitness

Clint's Insights

I used to think fitness was expensive…join a gym, hire a trainer, take time out of your day, etc. Well, after biting the bullet and making it a priority with my wallet and my calendar, I can say the time and money were well worth it. I realize that the "expensive" argument was just a head game I used as an excuse to not fully commit. And, the reality was that my unfit lifestyle cost me plenty. Those poor choices were not cheap. My perspective has changed. This side of the fitness track gives me the perspective that a strong body is a worthy investment.

Breah's Insights

When we first started our fitness program, I was on the scale a lot. I craved immediate feedback. If I had worked out so hard and been dieting all week, I wanted to see the results…tangible results. For me, at that time, the number on the scale had to be a certain number or I would be upset. I remember thinking to myself, "There is no way this is working because I am not seeing the number on the scale change." But it was working. Sometimes the number didn't move very much, but my clothes fit better, my body was more toned. The feedback was there—I just had to look in the mirror.

CHAPTER 8

Fitness B:
Get the Facts!

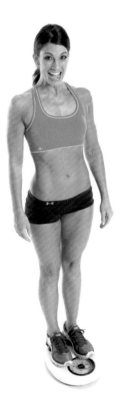

Before you read any further, go get your bathroom scale. Now, throw it out the window. Feel better?

Okay, you don't literally need to toss your scale out the window, but you do need to pack it away. The scale is not your friend. Addiction to a scale's reading can drive you in a negative direction. When you have worked really hard and the scale doesn't report the number you want, it will cause you to second guess the whole program. You'll come up with your own thoughts about how to lose weight. These are the same thoughts that have gotten you to the point that you picked up The Engagement Diet. So we have just one question: "How's that workin' for you?"

Ugh... Body Fat

One of the best fitness measurements is your percentage of body fat. Because you will be gaining lean muscle mass while losing body fat, the scale is a poor indicator of your true progress. If you're a woman who weighs 125 pounds and your body fat is 30%, this isn't good. One-third of your body is fat! If your body is a temple, you can hardly expect it to stay standing for a long time if it's built on a flabby foundation, even if the exterior looks good. For women, a total body fat percentage of 20 to 27 percent is a normal, healthy range. Women in great physical shape may have only 14 to 20 percent body fat. For men, 13 to 17 percent body fat is a healthy range, and with training, 10 percent is attainable. In this situation, the scale is not your friend. We have worked with many people who have worked out really hard for a week and stayed true to their eating plan only to have gained a pound. This is demoralizing, if you are using the scale as your measuring stick. Losing weight as indicated by the scale does not necessarily equate to being fit. How you look and how you feel is a better indicator.

One tool that doctors often use in lieu of the scale is the Body mass index (BMI). Body mass index is calculated by dividing a person's weight in kilograms by their height in meters squared. The U.S. Centers for Disease Control and Prevention traditionally consider an adult with a BMI between 25 and 29.9 as overweight, while an adult with a BMI of 30 or higher is considered obese. The one shortcoming of the body mass index is that it does not account for the weight of muscle vs. fat. Consequently, someone who is shorter and has a lot of muscle might have a BMI above 25 or 30 and still be in excellent shape.

Knowing your body fat percentage is a much better indicator of your physical

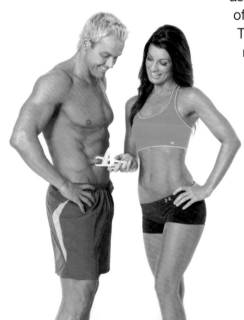

fitness and overall health. A body fat assessment is a very useful tool. As you become leaner your body fat percentage will drop. Knowing that percentage before you begin the program can help motivate you as well as give you an accurate starting point. Any local gym, as part of an initiation package, generally will perform the assessment for free. There are many methods of assessing body fat. Not all are 100% accurate; however, this is not as important as being consistent in using the same method when you begin and when you reassess to gauge your progress.

Which weighs more: a pound of fat or a pound of muscle?

As you burn fat you are building muscle. Fat does not turn into muscle and muscle does not turn into fat. They are two different types of tissue. But with The Engagement Diet, as you burn fat in your workout you are simultaneously building muscle. As you lose a certain volume of fat, you are adding a certain volume of muscle. They are in effect "replacing" one another. If the exact volume of space where you lost fat were replaced with the same volume of muscle, you would weigh more. Why? Because muscle weighs more than fat. Also, muscle has definition and fat does not. You can see the difference externally on your body.

The True Scale of Fitness

Another reason you won't need your bathroom scale for this program is that The Engagement Diet has its own scale. We call it the Jeans Scale. Don't most girls gauge their fitness level by how they look and feel in their "skinny" jeans? Guys might not admit it, but most have their favorite pair of denims, too. So, let's just use the universal scale—your jeans, something that everyone already has in their closet.

Here's what we suggest: From your closet (or your favorite jeans store) pick a pair of snug-fitting jeans (or pants). Put them on. These are your Phase I goal jeans. As your body reshapes itself, you will be able to tell that inches are coming off based on how your Phase I goal jeans fit.

At the end of four weeks you will be shocked at how those jeans fit. Believe it or not, they will fit nicely or even a bit loosely—one step closer to your goal. As a leap of faith and a statement that you trust the process, we would recommend two more things. At the same time you are picking out those snug Phase I goal jeans, we suggest you pick out two more pair of jeans in descending sizes. If your Phase I goal jeans are a size 12, buy a size 10 and a size 8 too. (For guys, if you are in a size 38, pick out a size 36 and size 34.) These are your Phase II and Phase III goal jeans respectively.

The Jeans Scale is much more reliable...and fun, we might add. Fitting into jeans you didn't even think you could get into is much more fun than believing the number on a scale that lies to you about your results. And if buying three pairs of jeans sounds extravagant, think of it this way: a good-fitting pair of jeans is an essential wardrobe item for both men and women. If you are getting fit for your big day and you are having half the success we expect you to have, then you will need new jeans. You don't want to attend your wedding functions in ill-fitting jeans. You want to look good. Buy the jeans and consider them multi-purpose: fashion statement and fitness scale.

Say Cheese

Unlike the scale, pictures don't lie. We recommend you take a picture of yourself each week to chart your progress. If you are like us, when you look in the mirror, you can't really register the physical changes you are experiencing. It's hard to notice the changes day to day as they relate to weight loss and fitness. At the beginning of each week take a picture of yourself, print it out and paste it in the spaces provided here in the book. You will have a living view of yourself over the course of the transformation. Week by week, this should motivate you as you see the progress.

Think about where you are now, and where you want to be. Cast a vision of what is possible. Put yourself there. Soak it up. Imagine every last detail of how it looks and feels to be in that space. Most people that pick up The Engagement Diet are looking to lose a few pounds before their wedding. Invariably along the journey they shift their thinking (and their goal) to being healthy. They get it. It is more about body fat composition than what the scale says. If my skinny clothes fit, then why should it matter how much I weigh? Don't get us wrong. You will lose weight. The point is that the weight loss as an end goal takes a back seat to the overarching fitness goals.

So, to summarize, your true measuring tools will be your body fat percentage, weekly photos, skinny jeans, and actual body measurements (e.g., waist, hips, etc.). You will find a helpful chart to track your measurements in the next chapter. Now let's get to it!

Fitness

Clint's Insights

Remember to put your workouts on your calendar consistent with your other appointments and obligations. When working out is on the calendar, it becomes a priority. When competing events or desires surface, you will be conscious about the trade-offs you are making given your priorities. You will find that if it is a priority, you will get it all done. Prioritize it and protect it.

Breah's Insights

The myth for women is that if you do any weight training you will build unsightly bulk. I had to overcome this myth myself, because girls don't want to look bulky. There is a difference between building muscle mass that provides lean definition and bulking up. The Engagement Diet is designed to provide women the definition they want, not bulk. I weighed 135 pounds and had 24% body fat when I started the program. By the twelfth week I was 125 pounds and 13% body fat. The scale did not reflect my true results. I lost two pant sizes and I was lean and toned. My body had completely reshaped itself. The results were clear.

CHAPTER 9
Fitness C:
Attack It!

Week one can be scary. You just have to start. Don't think, just start. When we started on week one, we didn't know what it would be like. We had the same questions as you do. We remember thinking that we'll believe it when we see it. We chose to focus on our excitement about what was possible and push the doubt to the recesses of our minds. When you do the program with someone else—especially someone you love—it gives you the energy to support one another. That's how we answered the question of why it was going to be different with this diet. Slowly we started to believe, and the power of unbelief began to loosen its stranglehold on us. Once we started listening to our trainer and we just did what he told us, everything started to change.

The Fitness Blueprint

We both came from families that weren't very fit. We grew up thinking that fit people don't smile, don't have fun, and they don't eat. Consequently, the tapes playing in our heads were not something to which we necessarily aspired. Whatever your family's relationship is to fitness and health, that is what you will believe. We want to change your way of thinking. Mesh your fitness blueprint to your spouse's blueprint. Choose to believe together that you can live differently and make healthy choices. Trust in your heart and mind that you are making a positive change. Trust that by getting fit, you will look better and feel better—and that by doing the program together, your commitment to each other will grow stronger. You can have a new relationship with fitness, and a new relationship with each other.

Statement of Goals

To know where you are going, you have to start with where you are. Establish a baseline for your current fitness level by taking some body measurements that will let you chart your progress. Take measurements in each of these target areas before you begin week one, and then measure each area again in week twelve. Trust us, you will want to know how many inches of fat were lost and how many inches were transformed into muscle.

Target Area	Week 1 Measurement	Week 12 Measurement
Waist		
Belly		
Hips		
Thighs		
Arms		
Chest		
Neck		
Calf		

The Voice in Your Head

Everyone has that voice in their head that plants seeds of doubt. We've experienced it, too. When we first committed to doing this program, that voice was loud. While we were able to silence it long enough to start, we wrestled with it continually. We know what it sounds like. As you choose to step out on the journey to fitness, we will coach you week to week on quieting that voice in your head so you can create the body—and life—that you love.

In working with other individuals and couples in recent years, we have observed that many people have a few things in common when it comes to their fitness goals. One of those things is that people rarely are accurate when it comes to self-evaluation. We are not able to see what others see in us. They see the truth and we often see untruths— lies that keep us from seeing what is possible. That voice in our head often sets us up to miss the opportunity for achieving our goals and living a life that we love.

We have put together a list of statements that the little voice in our head sometimes makes. Many may sound familiar to you. As you read them, evaluate whether the statement is a truth about who you are or whether it is an untruth you have just bought into over time. Next, ask yourself whether you can see past the statement to what is actually possible.

Girl Lies

- I'm the non-skinny girl who has never been in shape and probably never will be.
- I'm the former athlete or cheerleader who has let her weight slide.
- I'm getting older and just won't be able to attain the body of my earlier glory days.
- I'm the girl whose genetics preclude the possibility of being fit or even having any definition—just look at my parents.
- I'm the chronically poor eater who just can't stick to a healthy diet.
- I'm the girl who hates to sweat and doesn't feel comfortable at the gym.

- I'm the girl who is naturally thin and can eat anything and not gain weight. I don't ever work out, and I know I'm skinny fat.

Guy Lies

- I'm the chubby dude who is the life of the party but not in shape.
- I'm the high school or college athlete who stopped working out but didn't stop eating.
- I'm the hard-working professional with a growing belly. It just comes with the territory—look at everyone else in the office.
- I'm the guy who refuses to give up his favorite meals… they're just too good.
- I'm the guy who can eat five bowls of ice cream every night without gaining weight but gets winded walking across the parking lot.

There is no room for doubt or self-criticism in the fitness program. The Engagement Diet is all about positive change—it is about learning new habits to get healthy as a couple and entering into your marriage at your physical and emotional best.

Make it Easy on Yourself

Prepare for the week by getting the foods you need. Plan your days. Account for the events you have scheduled. Put clothes out the night before. Get your bottled water out.

Even in planning mode, you are working the program. When you fail to plan, you eat poorly and never go to the gym. If you are not prepared, then it is a lot easier to talk yourself into staying in bed. When you prepare in advance, you make it easier on yourself, because you don't let distracting thoughts pull you off course. You stay focused on the goal.

Ready? Then let's start the first week's workout!

Clint's Insights

When I finally committed to the program and stuck with it till the end, I awakened a sleeping giant. I realized there was a bad ass inside of me. This program ripped away everything except who I was at my core. I am so happy that I hung in there—that I didn't let my past belief of who I was ruin what was possible for me now. With each passing week it was a waning struggle. I know first-hand how hard it is to believe that it is possible, but at Week One that is all you can do: believe. You have to have faith. If you do the work, it is going to happen. Stay committed and the results will be there.

Breah's Insights

I never thought the program would work for me as a girl—especially the weight training. I had never really committed to anything like this. I worked hard to string together good choices each and every day. When I found myself making a bad choice, I acknowledged it and moved on. I recommitted. At the end of the whole process I noticed how powerful I was. This is not just about losing weight, it is about transforming my relationship to food, to fitness and with Clint. For me, it was a lifestyle change.

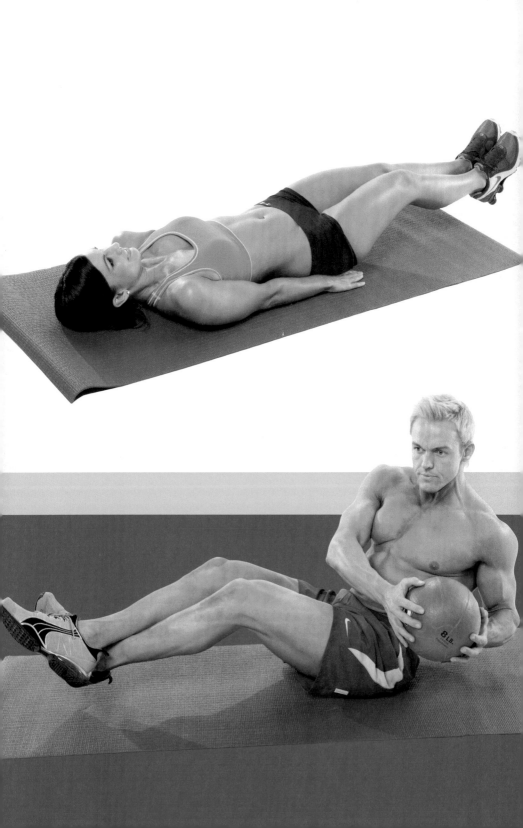

SECTION FOUR

FIT TO BE TIED IN 12 WEEKS

A Message from Breah

Ladies,

You are ready! You now have the tools to attack your diet and exercise. You can do this!

It is no accident that you are reading this book. You have chosen The Engagement Diet for a reason. Over the course of twelve weeks, you will have ups and downs, highs and lows. I assure you from personal experience you will come out of this having transformed yourself, your body and your relationship.

I know you have a lot going on right now. I have been there. I was shocked at the millions of excuses I came up with as to why this fitness thing could be put on hold—why I could focus on it another time. Think about completing this twelve-week program: it will be something that you will carry with you forever. It will be an even sweeter victory for having done it with your spouse. You guys will walk down that aisle and into your marriage as a true team. You will have the most powerful bond between you when you look into each others eyes and say "I do". Nothing could be better than that.

Clint and I had a level of commitment to one another after the program that I can hardly put into words. You just have to experience it for yourself. Trust me when I tell you this is meant to be. The outcome is beautiful. Put you and your spouse first for these twelve weeks so you can claim with confidence that you are fit to be tied.

Best,
Breah

A Message from Clint

Guys,

You have twelve weeks. Game on. You can see it, right? You know how great it can be. In your mind's eye, envision your future self. Grab hold of that reality and how great it will be for you and your fiancée. If you can do that, then you have all you need to be successful at the program. The time is now.

Choose to not let anything stand in your way. Silence that voice in your head. "I have all these things to do…what if she doesn't do it…" That voice in your head has nothing good to say at this point. Fear of what might happen in the future is not what is happening now. Seize the moment. The time is now.

Go get what you want. Be a leader for your home team. Your fiancée will love the strength of your choice. Who you are going to be for yourself and for your wife is over the top. Doing this program as a couple will lay a strong foundation for your entire marriage. The time is now.

If you stay committed to this program, I promise that you will transform yourself and your body. Your relationship will benefit immensely, too. Don't do what I did for so long when I refused to follow my trainers' instructions. Don't settle for just okay. The time is now.

I've got your back. It's only 90 days. I'll be with you the whole way. What do you have in the tank? Make this a priority. Push yourself. The other side is tremendous. This is it. Swing for the fence. Knock it out of the park.

Bring it!
Clint

WEEK ONE
Motivation:
The Choice Is Now

Congratulations—you're ready to start the program! It's always thrilling to choose something rewarding for yourself. Sometimes, though, we can lose sight of why we want to get fit and the benefits of making a positive change. Staying motivated is vital to achieving your goal. You are getting married...what great motivation! Your wedding day gives you every reason to stay on track. Focus on where you want to be—fixate on the end result. With motivation and support you can accomplish anything. If today you put on your clothes and you don't like how you look, you now have a plan to change that. You have a specifically tailored program to get you to where you want to be. With The Engagement Diet, you will feel great, look great in your pictures, and reflect back on the big day with pride.

YOU CAN DO IT

Maybe the idea of doing a twelve-week program is scary to you. Maybe you have tried a diet and fitness program before, but you didn't follow through. We are here to tell you, what is possible has nothing to do with the past. If you can imagine yourself at the end of the twelve weeks and truly get present to how that will feel, then you can do what you need to do. Every day is a choice. Life is a series of choices. At first, break the series down to the very next choice. Ask yourself, "What am I going to eat right now?" You don't have to be overwhelmed with the whole twelve weeks of choices. The NOW choice is the key in Week One.

During the next seven days, you will experience ups and downs. You will be tired and sometimes just flat out over it all. You will be pumped and your partner will be down, or vice versa. These feelings are part of the process. Any time you commit to something like this, you are not human if you do not feel challenged. Every morning when you get out of bed, commit that you will keep your word to yourself—just for that day. Stay true to your goal one day at a time, and at the end of the program you will be empowered with what you have accomplished. Just get started—take a step forward and see what happens.

YOU MIGHT BE ASKING:

Q: Do I really have time to do this right now, given that I have a wedding to plan?

A: In our experience, the reason most people don't have time is not because they have a wedding to plan. It is because fitness falls toward the end of their priority list. We say just choose. Choose to move it to the top of your priority list. If you have time for cake tasting and visiting the florist and selecting chicken or fish for the reception, you have time to go to the gym. The time issue will no longer be an issue as soon as you make your fitness an equal priority to your other responsibilities.

Q: What if my partner won't do the program with me? Or, what if my XO starts and then quits? I don't want to do this alone.

A: You are not alone. We are here for you as your coaches. More importantly, does it matter if your partner chooses not to participate? If you are waiting for both of you to be on the same page to do something, then you might miss the boat. Don't get us wrong—we are all about marital harmony and seeking unity on things. But at the end of the day you have to ask yourself, "Am I okay if my partner doesn't do it?" Whether or not your beloved participates really has nothing to do with you making a choice to do the program.

Ask yourself whether you are attached to your XO actually doing the program or whether you are committed to YOU doing the program. If you are attached to your partner doing the program and they choose not to do it, you are outsourcing your commitment. You are not making a commitment at all. Your commitment is contingent on some other factor beyond your control, namely your XO's choice whether or not to participate. When you are committed to your own health and fitness, then whatever your partner chooses does not change what you do. It is their choice—it's not about you.

Be supportive of whatever your partner chooses. You are on your way to the finish line. Congratulations!

WEEK ONE FOOD PLAN

21 meals + 14 snacks (Remember, your snacks should only fall in the Number 1 category)

- Number 1 meals – 14
- Number 2 meals – 5
- Number 3 meals – 2

Note: You can incorporate one extra snack per day if you find yourself needing that little extra fuel to make it through, but remember not to have more than three snacks a day.

WEEK ONE WORKOUT PLAN – Stir it up

Upper Body Circuit 30 min / **Cardio** 30 min — Monday, Thursday
Lower Body Circuit 30 min / **Cardio** 30 min — Tuesday, Friday
Abdominal Circuit 15 min / **Cardio** 45 min — Wednesday

Week One

RECOMMIT

Were you less-than-perfect your first week out? Everyone stumbles. The key is regaining your footing quickly and not letting the trip up lead to a complete fall. Acknowledge the things you didn't do compared to what you said you were going to do. Then, recommit. It is as simple as that. Common mistakes in Week One arise as a result of lack of planning or preparation. It's the first week of a brand new routine. Some things are not habits yet, but you'll get there. Recommit and move on to Week Two.

WEEK TWO
Doubt :
I Can't Do Anything

Doubt often starts to creep in at the beginning of Week Two. Sure, you made it through the first week, but can you really keep this up for the full program? If you say you can or you can't, you're right either way. You fail at everything you never try.

In our house, we try to nip doubt in the bud as soon as it rears its ugly head. Doubting whether we can do something is the opposite of our commitment—it is counter to what we have said we will do to make a positive change. Skepticism is inconsistent with our motivation and our goal of who we want to be.

Doubt messes with your mind. It is also contagious. We unwittingly use doubt to invite others into our underachieving mentality. We lure them in with comments, like, "I don't know if I can do it." When you are working the program together, this type of statement just pulls your XO down the rabbit hole with you. Doubters love company.

To combat doubt's insidious ways, we have dubbed it as selfish. When I say, "I doubt it will work," what I am really saying is that I want to quit or at least have the opportunity to quit at any time. This way, I don't really have to be accountable. I can blame the program and offer up excuses, like, "I'm too tired, I am sore, and I have to plan a wedding."

The words "I doubt" in effect reserve your right to do whatever feels good or tastes great. It is not useful. At the end of the day, doubt equals an unwillingness to give up control. Within the bounds of The Engagement Diet, it means unwillingness to let go of your unfit or unhealthy ways. Doubt precludes your ability to trust. Trust the process. What do you have to lose?

YOU CAN DO IT

Health and wellness are for everyone. If you trust the process the results will be there. This is universal. The program is based in science and nutrition—the results will be quantifiable.

When you stay committed for the long haul and come out on the other side, you empower yourself. The competition we were training for gave us a front row seat to the quitters' circle. Many gave up before getting to the finish line. Fear predominated. We were proud of ourselves for going through the process and sticking with it. We chose to let go and trust the program. We had each other the whole time to get through the tough parts, and the experience showed us how blessed married life was going to be. In the end, the euphoria was so great we wanted more. It is a lifestyle change.

You are probably still a little sore from Week One, and the food plan may be a big change from what you're used to, but in just one more week your body is going to start adjusting. Push through this week. By the time we get to next week you are going to start seeing results. Your clothes will feel different. Your eating will be more normal. The workout will just be part of what you do.

YOU MIGHT BE ASKING

Q: I'm tired and my muscles ache. Is this program too intense for me? Don't I need to rest?

Week Two

A: Aching muscles are a sure sign that the program is working! Tired and sore is exactly what you should feel. The first week of the program is designed to stir up your previously sedentary body. Your body may not be used to this much physical effort. Your muscles are talking to you. If you wait for them to no longer be sore before you head back to the gym, then the next time you work out you will experience soreness all over again. Soreness is caused by a build-up of lactic acid in the muscle tissue. The best way to get rid of that is to get back in the gym and continue your workout.

Q: I have to admit, I'm dying for a cheeseburger—but I'm afraid that my XO will think less of me if I own up to my weakness. If I slip up during the program, should I just keep mum?

A: If you change your actions based on what you assume another person's reaction will be, you will just end up resenting them. Get clear on your intentions—you are either committed to eating clean, or you are going to let yourself have a fun meal. If you choose a fun meal, then just choose it.

WEEK TWO FOOD PLAN

21 meals + 14 snacks (Remember, your snacks should only fall in the Number 1 category)

- Number 1 meals – 14
- Number 2 meals – 5
- Number 3 meals – 2

WEEK TWO WORKOUT PLAN – Stir it up

Upper Body Circuit 30 min / **Cardio** 30 min — Monday, Thursday
Lower Body Circuit 30 min / **Cardio** 30 min — Tuesday, Friday
Abdominal Circuit 15 min / **Cardio** 45 min — Wednesday

Week Two

RECOMMIT

With two weeks of data, you should see some patterns starting to emerge. For example, did you find that the day you pushed your workout off until the evening, it never happened? Do you default to the drive-through when you don't pack a lunch? Use this data to strategize and continue to set yourself up to succeed. Use the past to plan for the coming week. Focus on when it was easy and why. Identify what tripped you up. Then set yourself up for success.

Week Two

WEEK THREE
Comparison:
I Lose Every Time I Compare

You can always get the answer you want, if you tell yourself the right story. What story are you telling yourself? When I compare the inside of me to the outside of you, I lose every time. If you are comparing yourself to others—people in your family, at the office, at the gym— ask yourself about your motives. Are you trying to find inspiration or tear down someone else?

When you first start really getting fit, the urge to tear down those that are in really good shape can be strong. A part of you thinks, "If I'm not there yet, I don't want someone else to be there." The problem with that logic (or lack of logic) is that if you tear down something that you want, how can you get there? In effect, you are separating yourself from what you want—and that simply doesn't make sense.

YOU CAN DO IT

Human nature practically compels us to compare ourselves to others. It just happens. Most of the time, drawing comparisons is destructive to your overall goals. You are still at the beginning of the process. If you compare yourself to someone who is in better shape, you may have a hard time seeing how to get there. Then, if you are like us, you talk yourself out of even starting. In that regard, we become a Partner in Crime (PIC) and not an XO. We slowly start to convince ourselves—and our beloved—that the program isn't worth the effort, and that we'll never achieve the results we envision. Comparison leads to doubt, and doubt—if left unchecked—leads to failure.

This is where we say, "Check yourself before you wreck yourself." Recognize when you or your partner is being a PIC and not an XO. The PIC route is a slippery slope to failure for your goals. As soon as you notice comparison thinking, take that tantalizing opportunity to compare and make it positive. Let seeing others who are in great shape drive you to encourage one another and motivate you toward your goal. If you see others in a positive light, then your affinity for them and their achievements will grow.

YOU MIGHT BE ASKING

Q: I am hungry and I want a beer. My emotions are out of control. How do I deal with the stress of having to avoid foods and drinks that I really like but aren't part of the program?

A: Old habits die hard. While you think that you might never shake the urges or feelings you are having now, it will pass if you stick to it. Trust the process. Cling to the rock of your commitment. Get your personal letter out and read why you are choosing this. Shift your thinking from your current feelings to the big-picture motivation of why you began this journey. Re-enroll your XO. Communicate.

Q: This is supposed to be the most exciting time of my life, but I feel like I am depriving myself and missing out on all the fun that I should be having. How do I deal with the feelings of lack and achieve the perfect picture that I dream about?

A: Just when you made a choice to get on the right path related to your relationship with food and fitness, guess what shows up? Cupcakes. A steak dinner at the boss' house. Parties galore.

Temptation is inevitable. So are the feelings of deprivation that come with it. Up to this point, you have been choosing whatever you want. Although you didn't miss out on the cupcakes or parties, you did miss out on being the person you wanted to be as it related to your relationship with food and fitness.

Life is just a series of choices. What do you choose? Remind yourself of what you are getting and you won't be missing out. Think of your commitment to The Engagement Diet in the same terms as your commitment to love your spouse for the rest of your life. Is there someone else out there you are missing out on? No. What you gain by committing yourself to one person is the reward.

WEEK THREE FOOD PLAN

21 meals + 14 snacks (Remember, your snacks should only fall in the Number 1 category)

- Number 1 meals – 14
- Number 2 meals – 5
- Number 3 meals – 2

WEEK THREE WORKOUT PLAN – Stir it up

Upper Body Circuit 30 min / **Cardio** 30 min — Monday, Thursday
Lower Body Circuit 30 min / **Cardio** 30 min — Tuesday, Friday
Abdominal Circuit 15 min / **Cardio** 45 min — Wednesday

RECOMMIT

Did comparison trip you up this week? Comparison is a wicked friend. List the thoughts of comparison you have experienced this week. Write them all down on a sheet of paper. Now, tear it up. Burn it. Throw it in the trash. You are done with that. Take the energy you used to compare yourself to others and instead compare yourself to the best you. What is your potential? Go to that place and envision who you can be—who you *will* be. That is the comparison that will propel you toward your goals.

Week Three

WEEK FOUR

Me:
Living on the Fault Line

It is Week Four, and in case you forgot, this program is all about you. You are doing this for yourself. You are not doing The Engagement Diet for anyone else—not even your future spouse. You control your destiny in this program and in life, based on the choices you make. This week, tell yourself, "I choose ME."

Those of us who want to be helpful and focus on others have learned that until we make life about ME it can never fully or authentically be about others. The first step is to take responsibility for yourself. For example, in the first three weeks of the program, you can convince yourself that the choice of whether or not to do this program is about other people. You'll do it if your partner does it with you. You'll do it so your friends will comment on how great you look walking down the aisle. Those are perks, but they aren't the true reason you committed to the program. At the end of the day, you have to take responsibility for having made this choice for yourself.

That also means the success (or failure) rests solely with you. Do not outsource your achievements. Win or lose, you are not a victim of this program. Tell yourself, "The program doesn't have me, I have it." When you choose what you want, you will do it. The thoughts about "I should," or "I ought to" will not propel you to success. Make it about you—your choice.

YOU CAN DO IT

The "bad" news is that you are responsible for all things in your life. The good news is that if you are responsible for all things in your life, then you can change them.

If you are doing The Engagement Diet with your future spouse, be honest with each other. Be honest in your praise and honest when you slip up. Being real with one another is the power of the program. This epitomizes the relationship aspect of the program—permission to share with each other and support one another through the good days and bad. Practicing open, honest communication gives your partner the ability to offer their full support, even though you might have assumed you wouldn't receive it. Supporting one another drives you closer to each other. Support begets support.

This week is about staying focused on who you are in this program. Then you can begin to focus on who you are for each other. Listen to your XO this week. Take the time to learn how your XO needs support. Ask each other how you can best support one another. Do not speak out of judgment or condemnation. Your partner yearns for your love and encouragement. If you offer to listen, you are more likely to be heard in return. This is not about holding your XO accountable. Each of you is a valuable asset to the other. Learn to use one another to support the success you want to achieve individually and as a couple.

YOU MIGHT BE ASKING

Q: How do I stay consistent when my schedule is becoming increasingly hectic as we approach our wedding day?

A: Take it one week at a time. You don't have to worry about next month's consistency today. Just focus on one week at a time. If that is a challenge then just focus one day at a time. Break the time into the smallest increment on which you can train your focus. Week by week. Day by day. Hour by hour.

And don't forget to delegate. You don't need to do everything yourself. Who can you get to help you? You can't delegate your workout, so what can you delegate? Determine what you can pass along to others and delegate those tasks.

Q: I've messed up. I have been far from perfect with the program. How is that going to affect my results? I want to finish strong, but slip-ups make me question whether I have sabotaged myself to the point that I cannot achieve my goal.

A: Recommit. The fact you that you are asking this question demonstrates that your level of commitment is strong and that you are aware of your mistakes. Give yourself a break. This program is not designed for perfect people, because they don't exist. There is some margin for error. That is why we designed it with fun meals. You are human.

You can always recommit—any day, any time. Do what you can to make up for missteps. Do your workouts, eat clean, whatever it takes. Focus on what you can learn from the experience, both good and bad. That knowledge will fuel your journey. Every deviation can move you toward a fuller understanding of why you are doing the program.

One of our philosophies is that "life happens" and that the missteps are less of a big deal compared to the guilt related to those missteps and where that guilt could lead you. It is not necessarily the bad choice that is fatal. It is how you respond to that bad choice—what you choose to do afterward. What's done is done. You have the choice to move forward with the program. Say to yourself, "I choose ME."

Week Four

WEEK FOUR FOOD PLAN

21 meals + 14 snacks (Remember, your snacks should only fall in the Number 1 category)

- Number 1 meals – 14
- Number 2 meals – 5
- Number 3 meals – 2

WEEK FOUR WORKOUT PLAN – Stir it up

Upper Body Circuit 30 min / **Cardio** 30 min — Monday, Thursday
Lower Body Circuit 30 min / **Cardio** 30 min — Tuesday, Friday
Abdominal Circuit 15 min / **Cardio** 45 min — Wednesday

RECOMMIT

Now that you realize the program is about you, where can you push yourself? Remember the vision of your end goal. You are probably noticing that your clothes feel better. You are getting stronger. You are in the middle of planning your wedding, and still you are committed to change. Don't stress about the next eight weeks. Take the time to put yourself first and everything will work itself out. You are on your way. Own it. Phase I is complete. You've come through the toughest part mentally and set physical changes in motion. Enjoy the success you have achieved so far and get ready to build on it. Phase II will help you grow stronger physically, and it becomes more fun. The routine becomes a part of who you are and not just something on your to do list.

Week Four

WEEK FIVE
Compromise:
Beware of Creeping Doubt

"I'm more fit. I feel stronger. I look better. I rock. I've been doing awesome, so it's okay if I have an extra fun meal today. No biggie if I skip my morning workout. I'm already in better shape than I was before I started. Is it really that big of a deal?"

If you are asking yourself that question the answer is "Yes!" Be aware of the creeping effect of compromise. Your mind can start to play tricks on you. You question how you can make the program more comfortable and suitable for your life. You start to give some of the credit to yourself instead of the program. The trap of this thinking is that you feel so good you begin to believe you are the guru of your own fitness. You might begin to think:

- If I double up my workout I can make up for the one I skipped.
- If I do it myself I can get the same results.
- I am looking good so I can do whatever I want.
- I can relax a bit then really kick it in later and still be where I want to be in twelve weeks.

If adhering to the regimen of The Engagement Diet is not the sole cause of your success, there is room to change it without negative effects, right? Wrong! Don't compromise. Don't fiddle with the formula. You have the solution. Stick with it.

You still have eight weeks to go. You may have formed new habits, but the routines associated with your fitness and nutrition are still young and fragile. Don't jeopardize your success.

YOU CAN DO IT

To get the results you want, you've got to stick to the program. Less than a 100% effort yields less than 100% results. In life, sometimes "good enough" is enough, but at the end of the day, only you know what you really could have achieved, and where you fell short of giving it your all.

Choose to conquer this week. Keep your workouts a priority. You have a lot to do. You are very busy and it is stressful. The good news is, you don't have to reinvent the wheel. We have done the work for you. The program is all set for you to follow. Imagine yourself at twelve weeks. Stick with it. You will look awesome. You deserve this. Trust the program. Trusting the process means putting in 100% effort and letting the results speak for themselves. You will be amazed.

YOU MIGHT BE ASKING

Q: Why does the scale not reflect the progress I expect based on all the effort I have put in to this program?

A: The scale is not your friend. Do not invite it to the wedding. Save the postage. Go back to your goal. Society has brainwashed us to believe that scale = success. This is different. You are toning and transforming your body. You are building mass and muscle and reshaping your body. Weight is not a good measurement for this program.

To get a more accurate read on the progress you're making, take pictures of yourself each week or check your percentage of body fat.

It is empowering to see your body changing. Use that as your scale. Trust in the process. This plan works. When you look great on your wedding day, it won't matter how much you weigh.

Q: I can't help but feel skeptical. Will I really get the results I envision? I have done other programs and diets and they didn't work. Will this one really work?

A: You are on the way to getting lean and fit. This program is about being healthy. You are going to look amazing. This is a balanced workout and meal plan. The other programs you have tried may not have been as balanced. Doing this over time is going to give you a healthy beautiful sculpted body. Like a locomotive, it starts a little slow but once the machine is going, it is really moving with power. The momentum drives you forward toward a lasting lifestyle change. It is a long term effort, just like marriage.

WEEK FIVE FOOD PLAN

21 meals + 14 snacks

- Number 1 meals – 16
- Number 2 meals – 4
- Number 3 meals – 1

WEEK FIVE WORKOUT PLAN – Shape it up

Full Body Circuit 30 min / **Cardio** 30 min — Monday, Wednesday, Friday
Abdominal Circuit 15 min / **Cardio** 45 min — Tuesday, Thursday

RECOMMIT

Commit to yourself that the scale is not your friend. Find your true measurement. That could be your weekly picture or the way your skinny jeans fit. Whichever way you go, focus on that "scale" as the true assessment of your progress—your new measurement of success.

Week Five

WEEK SIX

Commitment:
My Word Is Like a Muscle

At the end of Week Six, you are halfway through The Engagement Diet. Some people discover that they are in better shape than in the recent past and tell themselves that the results are good enough— that they can roll with this and like it.

The question you should ask yourself is: when are you going to follow through on your commitment? You committed to the long term for the program in the same way that you are committing to the long term for your marriage. "Good enough" may be sufficient for the changes you are seeing in your body and your fitness. But the choices you make now are setting a precedent—a routine for how you will respond to many circumstances in your life. Quitting at the halfway mark sets you up for a roller coaster. When you're on a roller coaster, you don't go anywhere. You go up and down and in a circle, but there is no real transformation—no real progress.

Your word is like a muscle. You strengthen it by doing what you say you are going to do. What was your commitment to the program? When you commit to something, at first it's only your word. Then, actions begin. The evolution of your commitment is seen in the actions that are consistent with your word. At that point, you can really feel the level of your commitment —and even when you don't feel it, you can still rely on your word. It bridges the gap from your feelings to your actions.

Pushing through the desire to quit and actually sticking with the program is powerful. It sets the vision of who you are. You are either a person who fulfills your commitments or not. If your actions are based on your word (and not your feelings that day) you are demonstrating consistency, stability and honesty. People, including your XO, will believe you when you say you are going to do something. You are a person of character. Character matters. Marrying a person of character matters.

YOU CAN DO IT

When we begin to waver on our commitment, usually we want to get out of something. When we were preparing for the fitness competition, we found ourselves wavering on more than one occasion. We have learned that this wavering is a form of running from a breakthrough. What was really happening was that we wanted to eat and drink whatever we wanted. So instead of just eating badly (a fun meal) and giving ourselves a break, we went straight to rationalizing reasons to quit. Fortunately, we pushed through these emotions—we stuck to our word—and realized that, for us, "good enough" is not good enough when you are striving for *greatness.* If we had quit along the way, we would have always wondered, "What if? What would have happened if I had stayed committed? What could I have achieved?"

What is your commitment? When you started this program, you said you were going to do all twelve weeks. You are halfway there. Imagine yourself now in the twelfth week and how incredibly awesome it feels, in spite of the ups and downs along the way. Recognize that you stuck with it. You came through it with your XO. This vision will propel you through the remaining weeks of the program.

YOU MIGHT BE ASKING

Q: Some days, I'm really excited to hit the gym, and I've got a ton of energy. Other days, eating right and getting in my workout is a huge uphill battle. How do I get past the emotional slumps?

A: Motivation is a fickle thing—some days, you've got it in spades. Other days, it seems strangely absent. You don't feel like thinking about your food choices. You don't feel like working out. On those days, you have to "act your way into right thinking." In other words, sometimes you have to consciously choose to do what you know is best, even though you don't feel like it. Take the action first—choose the healthier meal, choose to get up early to hit the gym, choose to take the stairs instead of the elevator—even if you don't "want" to. The feelings will follow. As your body begins to take on a leaner, healthier shape and your stamina improves, you will find your motivation increases, too. You will want to stick with the program, because it works.

Q: I still am fearful about not reaching my goal. I am committed to the program, but now that I am halfway done, I am concerned I won't get there. How do I manage my fear?

A: Believe it or not, this feeling is completely normal. The urge to bail is a defense mechanism to avoid failure. Moreover, if you stick with the program and still don't get the results you want, someone has to be blamed. Will you blame us? Will you blame your XO? All these thoughts are part of the breakthrough. You are wrestling with who you want to be. Push through. Don't make this about us. Don't make it about your XO. Rest assured, you will get there. Believe it and continue doing the actions that demonstrate that you trust the process.

WEEK SIX FOOD PLAN

21 meals + 14 snacks

- Number 1 meals – 16
- Number 2 meals – 4
- Number 3 meals – 1

Week Six

WEEK SIX WORKOUT PLAN – Shape it up

Full Body Circuit 30 min / **Cardio** 30 min — Monday, Wednesday, Friday
Abdominal Circuit 15 min / **Cardio** 45 min — Tuesday, Thursday

RECOMMIT

Did you want to quit or slack off on the program? This is completely normal. Once we start seeing results, naturally we become our own expert. Stick with the program. The early results are there. Grab onto that success and find your new gear. Recommit mid-bite. Recommit mid-rep. This week, answer the question, "How can I push my fitness in the gym and my nutrition to the next level?" Make it a game.

WEEK SEVEN

Support :
True Support Comes from Me

Do you want to give unconditional love and total support to your spouse? Who doesn't? You want to be each other's XO. You want to support your partner without nagging. This far into the program, you may feel closer to your partner through the support that you give each other. Through trial and error, you may have figured out a language where you can support each other in a way that is uplifting and not condemning—and perhaps you discovered that sometimes, the best way to be supportive is to not say anything.

Marriage is a team sport. As a team, you are united—you are one. Choices are not about "his thing" or "her thing," but "*our* thing." The team is succeeding or losing, progressing or regressing, passing or failing. Through the program, we realize that we cannot truly live the life we love unless our XO is living the life they love. This is oneness. This level of support gives us the drive to kick things into another gear. We realize how the power of support can help us achieve our goals together as one.

YOU CAN DO IT

To succeed at your goal, both of you have to win. In this program and in marriage, you can't win if both of you do not win. That's the beauty of being one.

Give your partner space to learn how to be supportive. It is easy to make your XO wrong about how he or she is supporting you and start to wrestle with resentment. Remember, this is a learning process. Communication is key. Ask the right questions. "How do you like to be supported?" "When you ask me to hold you accountable, what does that look like?"

Sometimes, you have to be supportive even when it seems scary. Let your support be from your heart and not out of what you think your partner's support was to you. Give without expectation of receiving. If you want an awesome spouse, then be an awesome spouse. If you want support, then give support to your XO.

YOU MIGHT BE ASKING

Q: Do I really have time to learn how to be supportive of my XO on top of everything else I am doing? I thought this was a diet book. I am confused. Why do I need to also work on my relationship at the same time?

A: At the end of the day, you are doing a lot. You are preparing for a wedding. You are working out. You may be holding down a stressful job. If you are really going to do this program together, the relationship part is bound to come out. You each made a commitment—you are each making major lifestyle changes, and everyone has a different way of dealing with their emotions. Discovering how to support your XO will also open your eyes as to how you like to be supported. This, in of itself, is an amazing gift you can give one another.

Q: I know my XO is committed to the program, but they don't show support the way I would like. Sometimes, I feel like I'm flying solo. What should I do?

A: Doing the program with your future spouse can create a powerful bond between you, but you have to be honest with each other and share your feelings. Look for the right opportunity, and gently broach the topic by telling your partner how much their support means to you, and how much it helps you to stay motivated throughout the program. You may want to mention specific things that your XO could say or do that would really make a difference. When your XO shows support in the way that you like, affirm the gesture and say how much it means to you. And if they don't always deliver the encouragement that you need, offer some grace, and focus on lavishing your XO with love and support. Remember, your team is there to support you, too. Men and women communicate differently, and sometimes we need to lean on friends and family members for encouragement that really resonates.

WEEK SEVEN FOOD PLAN

21 meals + 14 snacks

- Number 1 meals – 16
- Number 2 meals – 4
- Number 3 meals – 1

WEEK SEVEN WORKOUT PLAN - Shape it up

Full Body Circuit 30 min / **Cardio** 30 min — Monday, Wednesday, Friday
Abdominal Circuit 15 min / **Cardio** 45 min — Tuesday, Thursday

RECOMMIT

Recommit to supporting your XO. Turn your mental attention to giving support. Let go of your expectation of the support you need. In marriage, showing grace for one another could be support your XO needs. Support for your XO comes from your listening to them and love for them. True support does not expect support in return. If you give support, it will come back to you.

Week Seven

WEEK EIGHT
Energy:
Bottled Up Desire

"I am getting fit, eating right and working on strengthening my relationship. Life is good. I have five weeks left and I feel strong in the gym and my food choices are transformed. I want to eat healthy. I embody fitness. That is who I am. I kick it in the gym. I like working out more than I thought I would. People are noticing my transformation. Some of these machines in the gym are mine. I own them. It is easier. We are working together rather than fighting each other."

If any of those statements resonate with you, then you are on the road to true transformation. Our word of caution during the euphoria of the moment is that you must be ever-vigilant to guard against backsliding. Why would we throw cold water on the jubilation of transformation? We want to see it complete. Our goal is that you experience lasting change.

YOU CAN DO IT

Life is like a heartbeat—it has a rhythm. You feel great right now. That is awesome. Chances are there will be a downbeat. Enjoy the journey. Make the most of it when you are on top of the world.

Minimize the downside when you are in the valley. Progress does not stop just because you are in the valley.

Life is a series of choices. Your new bad choices are not as bad as your old bad choices. We can easily forget the place from where we came. Get back in touch with that. See how far you have come. Pat yourself on the back. Recognize that you are being harder on yourself now because you can be. You now know what is possible.

When you are on your game, that is the time to find the next gear. What can you really do? You may be able to achieve a new level you might not have known was possible prior to the program. Go get it. You are shifting your norm to another level. Step up your game. Now is time to get even more out of the program and avoid a plateau. This is a pivotal point where you can choose to own it and make it yours. Your body knows you have more in the tank. Do more. You rock!

YOU MIGHT BE ASKING

Q: I feel great about what I have achieved, and now I'm worried about our honeymoon. It's supposed to be all about fun and relaxation, but I'm concerned that if every meal is a fun meal, I'm going to regain the weight and reverse all the progress I made. How can I enjoy our honeymoon without sabotaging myself?

A: Now that the program has become a way of life, you can find a happy medium when you're on vacation. For example, just because you're not going to be as stringent as eating all Number 1 meals every day doesn't mean that the alternative should be only fun meals. Focus on Number 2 meals, which are still a fair choice. Have one glass of wine instead of three. Look for opportunities to work out that may not involve going to a gym, like running on the beach, swimming at the hotel pool, or taking a walking tour of the town or city you're visiting on your honeymoon.

Q: I have worked really hard to follow the formula you present in the book, and I feel great. How can I take the program to the next level?

A: Have you increased the weights you are using during the routine? Have you shortened the rest time between reps? Are you doing the program full out? Some suggestions: Utilize the help of a trainer to suggest a more intense workout...substitute some Number 1 meals in place of some Number 2 and 3 meals. Most of all, just continue doing the program and your body will continue to transform. As you become stronger, you will be better able to "take it to the next level."

WEEK EIGHT FOOD PLAN

21 meals + 14 snacks

- Number 1 meals – 16
- Number 2 meals – 4
- Number 3 meals – 1

WEEK EIGHT WORKOUT PLAN - Shape it up

Full Body Circuit 30 min / **Cardio** 30 min — Monday, Wednesday, Friday
Abdominal Circuit 15 min / **Cardio** 45 min — Tuesday, Thursday

RECOMMIT

You are on your way. Recommit if you had any trip-ups this week. Recommit to your diet, workout, and your relationship. Use this week as an imprint of what your new normal feels like. Lock it in. Tap into it when you don't remember what awesome feels like. Staying in touch with that feeling will fill your motivation tank for years to come.

Week Eight

WEEK NINE

Transformation:
What It Really Means to Feel Good

You have transformed. When you used to say you felt good, you didn't really even know what feeling good meant. Now you do! Do you recognize it? It is who you are. We say, "It is who you BE." You feel it. It is not hard work anymore, right? You have experienced a mental shift. You have started to desire the effects that eating right and working out bring to your daily life. It is a new normal, the "real" feeling of feeling good.

Fitness and sound food choices have gone from something that you do to part of who you are. The way in which people now relate to you is encouraging and inspiring. Your default state used to be an unhealthy lifestyle, and now your default state is to make healthy choices. You're not just doing a program; you are changing your lifestyle.

YOU CAN DO IT

You have a new relationship to food. You have a new relationship to fitness. You have a new relationship with your XO. The old is gone and the new is here. Transformation. Hooray!

Ironically, some people don't want you to be the new transformed you. They want you to be the old you. They want to have the old relationship with you. Our experience is that some people will even go so far as to squash your possibilities. They want to pull you back into old habits and behaviors—into the old way of being.

We use the tribal energy of our relationships to really determine the things to which we are committed. When you understand how others may want to sabotage your efforts, you can prepare a strategy for handling those situations. You don't have to buy into their way of thinking. Just relish the knowledge that you are transformed. Some may relate to you as the old you. You know you have changed. Your XO knows it, too. Physically and mentally, you are reaching new heights. It's okay if others don't get it. Let them adjust in their own time.

YOU MIGHT BE ASKING

Q: This may seem silly, but I'm afraid to throw away my old clothes. I've already dropped two sizes, but I have a hard time believing it will last. Should I keep my big jeans for after the wedding?

A: Holding onto your big jeans means you're holding onto bad habits—you're leaving the door open to backslide in the future. Focus on what you have achieved, and celebrate it. Embrace it—lock it in and understand that you don't have to go back. You always have a choice.

Q: How hard will I have to work to maintain the results I have achieved to this point? If I don't work this hard all the time, will my results evaporate?

A: The program's level of intensity is for a certain milestone level of fitness. It is not the level of intensity needed to maintain your results. One bad choice in one day is not going to automatically take you back to your prior unhealthy state. You can down-shift into third gear and still maintain the level of fitness you've achieved. Remember, diet is 80% of your results. You can maintain a healthy lifestyle by hitting the gym for 60-90 minutes three times per week and eating a clean diet.

Week Nine

WEEK NINE FOOD PLAN

21 meals + 14 snacks

- Number 1 meals – 18
- Number 2 meals – 2
- Number 3 meals – 1

WEEK NINE WORKOUT PLAN - Dial it in

Full Body Circuit 45 min — Monday, Wednesday, Friday
Abdominal Circuit 15 min — Monday, Wednesday, Friday
Cardio 1 hour — Tuesday, Thursday

RECOMMIT

This is what you wanted before you started. You are in the home stretch. Stay focused. Push yourself harder. Make sure you always have a plan in place, so you set yourself up to succeed. Make a plan every week—every day—to put yourself first. Plan your meals. Plan your workouts. Make these last three weeks more powerful than anything you have experienced so far. Don't settle. Discover what is possible for your big day. Keep going. You deserve it.

Week Nine

WEEK TEN
Powerful:
Inside the Real Me

"It's free" is rarely a good excuse for breaking your commitment and losing the powerful effect of your hard effort.

Are you powerful? Do you choose to be powerful? If you are eating poorly, can you stop? You might think you can't stop, but you can. We used to think that once the seal was broken on a bad choice, we had to give in. If I eat one chip (unhealthy choice), I have to eat the whole bag. You can recommit whenever you want. Just because you eat poorly the first meal of the day does not mean you have to eat badly the rest of the day. Don't beat yourself up; give yourself a break and get back on track. At any point you can choose to stay committed.

YOU CAN DO IT

You can choose to recommit whenever you want: mid-bite, mid-meal, mid-day, mid-vacation…You get it!

At the Mexican restaurant, we ended up choosing not to eat the bad stuff even though it was free. Just because something is free doesn't mean it tastes better. Although the *queso*, margaritas and *sopapillas* that the waiter delivered might have been a temptation before, we were in Week Ten of the program, and we were committed. We sent it all back. We were saying no from a place of power.

Even though you are feeling super powerful, you still may find yourself putting a cookie to your mouth once in a while. But you're no longer just following your habit. Now you catch yourself and rethink your actions. Something powerful happens when you step away mid-choice. Sticking to your word and making a different choice is a sign of your inner strength. You have a new tool in your bag of tricks.

At some point you are going to want to have a cookie and you are going to have a cookie. That's okay, but you can still choose to go back to your original commitment. Give yourself grace and get back on it. Stay on track. If you make a bad choice, own it and move on.

YOU MIGHT BE ASKING

Q: This program has been such an incredible experience— how can I share this with others?

A: Is there anyone for whom you might be an example? To influence others, focus on the people who are reacting positively to you regarding your fitness. These are the ones who are curious. They are open to what you have to share. Realize the impact you are having and just keep going. Finishing strong is the best way to influence others.

Q: I am fully committed, but this program is causing problems in some of my relationships. What do I do?

A: People are funny. They will react in ways that you do not expect. Stay focused on the fact that this is your deal. Their reaction to you doing this program is not a reflection on you—it more likely has to do with their own challenges and feelings about commitment or how relationships should be. Roll with it. Love them where they are and stay focused. It is okay to do something just for you.

Week Ten

WEEK TEN FOOD PLAN

21 meals + 14 snacks

- Number 1 meals – 18
- Number 2 meals – 2
- Number 3 meals – 1

WEEK TEN WORKOUT PLAN - Dial it in

Full Body Circuit 45 min — Monday, Wednesday, Friday
Abdominal Circuit 15 min — Monday, Wednesday, Friday
Cardio 1 hour — Tuesday, Thursday

RECOMMIT

You have two weeks left. Believe it or not, a lot can change in the last two weeks. You built an engine. Use it. Challenge yourself. Eat only Number 1 meals. Focus on fuel. Push that extra ten percent during your workout just to see how great your results can be. Do something loving for your XO to show your support. Sprint toward the finish line! Your big day is almost here!

Week Ten

WEEK ELEVEN
Unstoppable:
I Am Bulletproof

You are two weeks from finishing the program, and your wedding is just around the corner. When you started this program, we encouraged you to envision yourself in this place. Here you are. Love yourself for what you have accomplished, and who you have become for you and your future spouse. You have an incredible physique and a great relationship as you head into your marriage. Take time to reflect. Think about your big day. Take it all in. You have given yourself a gift that keeps on giving. Take your food, fitness, and relationship to the next level this week. You are unstoppable.

YOU CAN DO IT

Be unstoppable. Bulletproof, indomitable, unbeatable, and invincible. The choice is yours. The program transformed us. Now you are transformed. Just knowing this makes you unstoppable. It is real. You have the tools. You choose to do it or choose not to do it. Fitness and nutrition no longer just happen to you. You are responsible for your choices. It's a lifestyle change.

The rest of this program is a breeze. Keep knocking it out. Smart food choices are key. You will still achieve another level before your wedding day. Stay with the food plan. It will get you where you need to be. The bonus is that you and your partner are in great shape. You will have a great time on your honeymoon. Cheers!

YOU MIGHT BE ASKING

Q: How do I really make sure that this becomes a lifestyle change and I don't fall back into bad habits?

A: You have the choice. You have probably picked up on this theme by now. Choose it. Only you can choose whether the program was a one-time fluke or a new way of living.

Q: Can I choose to continue this way of life and still have fun?

A: Absolutely. One key is that, as you adopt new habits, you will find that you have a new definition of "fun." Is it more fun to scarf down an entire pizza or to feel great about the way you look in your skinny jeans? Is it more fun to get an extra hour of sleep in the morning or to have enough energy to tackle anything that life throws at you because you start the day with a sixty-minute workout? Continue to answer the question, "Who do you want to be?" Reaffirm who you are in the realm of "fun" given your new good choices. Choose the long-term fun of being fit and looking great!

WEEK ELEVEN FOOD PLAN

21 meals + 14 snacks

- Number 1 meals – 18
- Number 2 meals – 2
- Number 3 meals – 1

WEEK ELEVEN WORKOUT PLAN - Dial it in

Full Body Circuit 45 min — Monday, Wednesday, Friday
Abdominal Circuit 15 min — Monday, Wednesday, Friday
Cardio 1 hour — Tuesday, Thursday

RECOMMIT

What tripped you up this week? Probably nothing. You rocked it. You are feeling what it's like to summit the mountaintop. What you once thought was the top of your fitness potential has now become your bottom—the minimum you expect from yourself. At this place, there is no recommitment needed. You are committed. Your fitness level now has a new norm. Remember when we asked you to put yourself in this place during week one? Be with it. You are here! How does it feel? As your life waxes and wanes, you can draw on those feelings and use them as motivation when you want to reach for that mountaintop again. You rock!

WEEK TWELVE
Love:
My Light Is Shining Brightly

We are so proud of you guys. You should be proud of yourselves, too. This is a big deal. You committed to this program twelve weeks ago. You stuck with it. You traveled the ups and downs of the journey.

Let the light of this moment shine bright. You are probably only days away from your wedding. Throughout this book we have attempted to give you encouragement and guidance as you developed a new relationship to food, fitness and your XO. You no longer need us to stand for you in that. You can stand for yourself. Congratulations.

WEEK TWELVE FOOD PLAN

21 meals + 14 snacks

- Number 1 meals – 18
- Number 2 meals – 2
- Number 3 meals – 1

WEEK TWELVE WORKOUT PLAN - Dial it in

Full Body Circuit 45 min — Monday, Wednesday, Friday
Abdominal Circuit 15 min — Monday, Wednesday, Friday
Cardio 1 hour — Tuesday, Thursday

YOU CAN DO IT

What you have done is big. When you play big, the people around you get to play big. Minimizing your greatness robs others of the encouragement to play big. Play big! Take the time to congratulate yourself. Soak it up. Be proud and stand proud. YOU DID IT!

Week Twelve

EPILOGUE

A Message for the Groom

I am stoked that you completed the program! You committed and your relationship to food and fitness has transformed. I am proud of you. I know it was a ton of work, and now you have come full circle. When I started getting serious about fitness, I was focused on having a better body. Through doing the program with my XO, I ended up honing my skills of commitment. I use it in my marriage every day. As you prepare to make the biggest commitment of your life, know that you have strengthened that muscle of commitment for the past twelve weeks. Your word is strong. The commitment that it takes to get through the program is exactly the commitment to get through marriage. You make one choice after another with the goal of always being your best, and of supporting your XO to the max.

In marriage you are the leader. For most of my single life, my choices affected me alone, but when I got married they affected both my wife and me. This was a big responsibility, but an awesome one. Make good choices and have grace with your wife. Listen. Listen. Listen. Then talk. My wish for you is that you will always love and protect your wife like you did when you first met.

My toast to you on your wedding day is that you pursue your relationship with your wife with the fullest commitment throughout your life. Her love should always be your number one pursuit.

Your buddy,
Clint

A Message for the Bride

You are about to embark on your first year of marriage and you will find yourself using things you have learned in this program every day. Using these tools is a choice. Some days you may question whether the program is still working for you. Remember that you are powerful individually and as a couple. You can create your own reality through the power of your commitment.

Marriage is one of the most rewarding things in my life. It is not the easiest. This book was inspired because of our desire to love and support one another. My gift to you is the encouragement to be true to yourself. You are a beautiful person inside and out. You did this! I am proud of you. Be powerful and responsible for your choices in life. Congratulate yourself when you do well and laugh at yourself when you mess up. Toast your failures that give you the perspective to see the true successes. Love, respect and honor your spouse to give him confidence to lead you in this journey called life. Own your greatness. Demonstrate unconditional love for everyone in your life so they can shine as brightly as you.

Love,
Breah

APPENDIX

QUICK PICK™ MEAL PLAN BY NUMBERS

Weeks	#1 Meals	#2 Meals	#3 Meals	Snacks
1 to 4 Phase One	14/week	5/week	2/week	14/week (2/day)
5 to 8 Phase Two	16/week	4/week	1/week	14/week (2/day)
9 to 12 Phase Three	18/week	2/week	1/week	14/week (2/day)

Remember: Your body is like a furnace, and your metabolism burns the fuel that you put inside. You can burn energy more effectively when you feed the fire throughout the day with several smaller meals and snacks, rather than eating a huge meal (a big log) that will put out the fire. That feeling of being in a food coma after you eat a huge meal is evidence of the way it shuts down your system. Small meals keep that metabolism up and burning those calories.

If you want to really dial it, then just drop your Number 3 meals during the last two weeks to really turn up the heat.

Meals

Phase I – Quick Pick™ Meal Plan

During the first four weeks, you are learning the ropes and learning which foods fall into which meal category. Use the chart below to create a roadmap for the week to help you stay on track with your food choices.

21 meals + 14 snacks (Remember, snacks are only in the Number 1 category)

- Number 1 meals – 14
- Number 2 meals – 5
- Number 3 meals – 2
- Snacks – 14

Note: You can incorporate one extra snack per day if you find yourself needing that little extra fuel to make it through, but remember not to have more than three snacks a day.

Here is an example of one way to organize your meals for the week, but you can plan your meals any way you choose. We prefer to put most of our Number 2 and Number 3 meals on or near the weekend when we are more socially active with friends and family. During the week when we are back in our routine we focus more on Number 1 meals.

	Sun	Mon	Tue	Wed	Thu	Fri	Sat
Breakfast	2	1	1	1	1	1	2
Snack	1	1	1	1	1	1	1
Lunch	1	1	1	2	1	1	2
Snack	1	1	1	1	1	1	1
Dinner	1	1	2	1	1	3	3
Snack	1	1	1	1	1	1	1

Phase II – Quick Pick™ Meal Plan

At this point, you start to get it. You can begin to play with your food (figuratively) and get into a routine.

21 meals + 14 snacks

- Number 1 meals – 16
- Number 2 meals – 4
- Number 3 meals – 1
- Snacks – 14

Here is an example of one way to organize your meals for the week, but you can plan your meals any way you choose by simply inserting the correct amount of Number 1, 2 and 3 meals in your plan for the week.

	Sun	Mon	Tue	Wed	Thu	Fri	Sat
Breakfast	2	1	1	1	1	2	1
Snack	1	1	1	1	1	1	1
Lunch	1	1	1	1	2	1	1
Snack	1	1	1	1	1	1	1
Dinner	1	1	2	1	1	1	3
Snack	1	1	1	1	1	1	1

Meals

Phase III – Quick Pick™ Meal Plan

You are dancing on the edge of a lifestyle change. You will feel the breaking of any addictions to food you might have had. A new relationship to food is on the horizon!

21 meals + 14 snacks

- Number 1 meals – 18
- Number 2 meals – 2
- Number 3 meals – 1
- Snacks – 14

Here is an example of one way to organize your meals for the week, but you can plan your meals any way you choose by simply inserting the correct amount of Number 1, 2 and 3 meals in your plan for the week.

	Sun	Mon	Tue	Wed	Thu	Fri	Sat
Breakfast	1	1	1	1	1	1	1
Snack	1	1	1	1	1	1	1
Lunch	1	1	1	2	1	1	1
Snack	1	1	1	1	1	1	1
Dinner	2	1	1	1	1	1	3
Snack	1	1	1	1	1	1	1

Meals

For more tips, tools and information about The Engagement Diet, please visit our website at www.theengagementdiet.com.

QUICK PICK™ FOOD LIST

Over the duration of the program you will go through three phases. Each phase is made up of four weeks. Each week is made up of thirty-five meals, which represents five meals a day. That may sound like a lot, but two of the "meals" each day should be only snacks designed to help stave off major hunger pangs and rev up your metabolism. Some of you may find that you need a little extra fuel to get through the day, so we recommend that you simply add one extra snack into your diet on those days you really need it.

Here is the list of food items broken down into Number 1 and Number 2 categories.

Number 1 Food List

PROTEIN

Cod	Tilapia
Egg whites	Tuna
Orange roughy	Turkey
Salmon	White chicken
Sea bass	

COMPLEX CARBS

Arugula	Cream of rice
Asparagus	Cucumbers
Black beans	Green beans
Broccoli	Green peas
Brown rice	Greens (salad)
Brussels sprouts	Oatmeal
Carrots	Spinach
Cauliflower	Sweet potato
Celery	Zucchini

Meals

SNACKS

1 tbsp almond butter
Blackberries
Blueberries
Broccoli
Carrots
Celery
Cranberries (unsweetened)
Cucumber
Grapefruit
Greek yogurt (add protein powder and sugar substitute)

Green apples
Greens (salad)
Oatmeal
Raspberries
Raw almonds
Small piece of protein
Spinach
Sweet potato
Flavored high-grade protein powder shake
Zucchini

SPICE IT UP

Ketchup
Mustard
Peppers
Pickles
Salsa
Salt
Pepper

Use: Cooking spray instead of oil or butter

Add: Tomatoes, mushrooms, onions, spinach, etc. to egg whites or ground turkey

DRINKS

Coffee
Tea (hot or cold)
Diet soda
Light sugar-free drink
Water or sparkling water

Meals

Example Number 1 Meals

Remember, your ideal meal will be a hand-size portion of lean protein (think chicken or fish), a fist full of complex carbohydrates (think broccoli or sweet potato), and a thumb-size portion of fat (like avocado, nuts, olives, or almond butter), which helps to lubricate the digestion.

This method makes it very easy to measure your food without having to whip out of your back pocket a scale or measuring cups and spoons. We specified cups and ounces in the examples below, but that is just for a frame of reference.

BREAKFAST

1/2 cup to one cup of cooked oats with handful of blueberries
1 piece of turkey bacon
Coffee, black or with artificial sweetener

Egg white omelet with tomatoes, onions, and spinach
1/2 cup to one cup cooked oats, plain or with flax seed
Iced tea, plain or with artificial sweetener

2 scrambled egg whites
2 pieces of turkey sausage
1/2 cup to one cup of cream of rice with handful of raspberries
Hot tea, plain or with artificial sweetener

LUNCH

Turkey breast (6-8 oz) with one cup of brown rice
Light sugar-free drink or water

Grilled chicken breast (6-8 oz)
Cup of mashed sweet potatoes
Sparkling water

Seared tuna salad w/ clear nonfat dressing
Cup of brussels sprouts
Iced tea, plain or with artificial sweetener

Meals

DINNER

Grilled chicken (6-8 oz) salad with clear nonfat dressing
Diet soda

Grilled chicken breast (6-8 oz)
Cup of cauliflower
Iced tea, plain or with artificial sweetener

Grilled tilapia (6-8 oz)
Cup of broccoli
Water

SNACKS:

Green apple with1 tbsp of almond butter
Grapefruit with artificial sweetener
Greek yogurt with a scoop of protein powder and artificial sweetener

Remember: NOT ALL CARBS ARE CREATED EQUAL! Simple carbohydrates are broken down quickly and easily converted to fat. Examples of simple carbs include tortillas, chips and breads. Complex carbohydrates are broken down more slowly and allow the body to burn them off, minimizing their conversion to fat. Examples of complex carbs include broccoli, green beans, and leafy green vegetables.

Number 2 Food List

PROTEIN

Lean red meat (filet mignon, New York strip)
Deli meat
Pork chop

CARBS

Pinto beans
Wheat pasta

White potatoes (plain)
White rice
Whole grain bread

Adding a small portion of these items will turn your Number 1 meal into a Number 2 meal:

Bananas	Pears
Cashews	Pecans
Grapes	Pistachios
Oranges	Plums
Peaches	Walnuts
Peanuts	1 tbsp. peanut butter

Example Number 2 Meals

BREAKFAST

Egg white sandwich on wheat bread
Cup of fruit
Coffee, black or with artificial sweetener

2 eggs over easy
1 piece turkey sausage
Wheat toast
Water

LUNCH

Turkey sandwich on wheat with mustard and veggies (no cheese)
Iced tea, plain or with artificial sweetener

Grilled chicken fajitas with thumb-sized portion of guacamole (no tortillas)
Side salad with clear nonfat dressing
Diet soda

Meals

DINNER

Turkey with whole-wheat spaghetti pasta in light marinara sauce
Iced tea, plain or with artificial sweetener

6-8 oz filet of lean red meat
Baked potato
Iced tea, plain or with artificial sweetener

SNACKS

There are no Number 2 snacks. Refer to your Number 1 snack list for all your daily snacks.

For more tips, tools and information about The Engagement Diet, please visit our website a www.theengagementdiet.com.

QUICK PICK™ FOOD TIPS

1. Shop for your food on Sundays. This gives plenty of time to plan your meals and get your food prepared for the week.

2. Use our grocery list. It has all the food to make an infinite number of Quick Pick™ meals categorized by grocery store section. Place it on your fridge each week and check what you need as you go. When Sunday rolls around, you are ready to shop for what you need.

3. Make meals to go. Protein bars and shakes are good portable meals. Almonds are another easy on-the-go option.

4. Cook your food in advance. We like to cook our proteins (e.g., chicken, lean cuts of steak) and use them throughout the week. Our veggies get chopped and put in steamer bags. We just drop them in the microwave and a few minutes later we have a great meal.

Meals

5. Use our weekly planner to budget your Quick Pick™ Meals by category: Number 1s, Number 2s and Number 3s. Identify work lunches and wedding dinners first so you can plan around them.

6. List your favorite fast food restaurants. Go online and research their menus. Find your new favorite meal according to your food goals and stick with it when you feel the need to drive through.

7. Portion control is the name of the game. Protein at your meal should not exceed the size of your hand.

8. When eating out, don't use the menu. Don't even look at it. Decide what you want before you open the menu with its pictures of T-bone steaks, hearty mac and cheese and hot fudge layer cakes.

9. Pack your snacks in single serve plastic bags. Place them at every location you will be during the day or carry them with you; e.g., your car, office, gym bag, etc.

10. Don't be boring. Pick a variety of foods. Change it up. Plan for variety so you don't find yourself in a rut.

11. Plan your treat meals. Wedding activities will cause a busy social calendar. Take the stress out of it by planning those Number 3 meals in advance.

12. You're doing this together. Use that to your advantage. Eat together. Be together. Share your successes and struggles. Support good eating habits.

13. De-bulk. Often bulk stores have only those foods that can be sold in bulk, which are typically Number 3 foods. Eat less and spend more on quality food.

14. Steer clear of processed foods. Don't walk the interior of the market. Shop the perimeter, where you'll find fruits, vegetables, meats, eggs and dairy.

Meals

15. Highly processed foods equal long shelf life, so if the food can last a long time either in the fridge or pantry, it's probably not a good choice.

16. When selecting proteins, choose free range over caged or farm-raised, and wild fish versus farm-raised fish. Avoid protein raised on steroids or hormones.

17. Fruits and veggies are "all natural". Some are simple carbohydrates and others are complex. Complex carbohydrates are a better choice because the body breaks them down more slowly in processing them for fuel. That means there is a less likelihood of the carbs turning to sugar and being stored in your body as fat.

18. Artificial sweeteners keep calorie counts lower. Pick the one you like and keep it handy for your coffee, yogurt snack or oatmeal.

19. Cut back on sodas. Don't drink your calories. Coffee and tea (natural caffeine) are okay. Just watch the sugar as a sweetener.

20. Water, water, water. Drink half your weight in ounces. If you weigh 200 pounds, you should drink 100 ounces of water.

21. Alcohol is basically sugar as it relates to your body chemistry. We say, "don't drink" during the program. For some of you, that is not realistic, given the wedding planning season. So if you drink, clear liquors (e.g., vodka, gin) and red wine will have the least negative impact to your diet. Rum, tequila and whiskey are next on the list. The worst choices are brown liquors and white wine.

22. Have a glass of wine then a glass of water. Alternate your consumption, so you can pace yourself in social settings.

23. If you find yourself in social settings and you just don't want to hassle with a lot of questions, you can always

order sparkling water with lime. People will naturally think it is a cocktail.

24. When drinking, be conscious of the portion. A glass of red wine does not mean a goblet of red wine.

25. Try serving your new smaller portions of food on a smaller plate. Even though you plated it, you will be surprised how your mind tricks you into perceiving a full plate of food.

26. Try eating slower. Enjoy your meal. Give yourself time to feel the fullness that you are giving your body with the proper food and correct portions.

27. Eat with your partner. Minimize the huge portions offered at restaurants by splitting a meal. If you are having a fun meal, just split the cheeseburger.

28. Foods to avoid include dairy products (cheese, yogurt, whole milk), creamy condiments like mayonnaise and ranch dressing, and simple carbs (chips, tortillas, white bread, pasta).

29. Juices can have a lot of sugar. Try unsweetened fruit-flavored tea or sugar-free drink instead.

For more tips, tools and information about The Engagement Diet, please visit our website a www.theengagementdiet.com.

Meals

FITNESS ABC GUIDE

Weeks 1 through 4: "Stir it up"

MONDAY/THURSDAY

Upper Body Circuit 30min/High Intensity Interval Training (HIIT) Cardio 30min

Note: Always stretch 6-10 minutes before performing any exercise routine. We do not recommend starting any workout routine without first doing some type of warm up.

Upper Body 30min, 3-6 circuits/sets of each

Circuit: each circuit consists of performing one exercise for each muscle group 12-15 reps, then moving immediately to the next exercise. The circuit is complete when all muscle groups have been worked. Upper body circuit consists of the following muscle groups. Example exercises can be found in the Fitness ABC Training section in the following pages.

1. Chest
2. Back
3. Shoulders
4. Biceps
5. Triceps
6. Abs

High Intensity Interval Training (HIIT) Cardio/30min

High Intensity Interval Training (HIIT): choose a cardio machine such as treadmill, bike, elliptical or stair climber and start with a 5-minute warm-up at low intensity, then for 20 minutes alternate between high and low intensity for 30 second to one-minute intervals. Then finish with 5 minutes of cool-down. To keep it interesting, you can always switch from one machine to the next during your 30-minute cardio.

Training

TUESDAY/FRIDAY

Lower Body Circuit 30min/High Intensity Interval Training (HIIT) Cardio 30min

Lower Body 30min, 3-6 circuits/sets of each

Circuit: each circuit consists of performing one exercise for each muscle group 12-15 reps, then moving immediately to the next exercise. The circuit is complete when all muscle groups have been worked. Lower body circuit consists of the following muscle groups. Example exercises can be found in the Fitness ABC Training section in the following pages.

1. Lunges
2. Squats
3. Leg Extension
4. Leg Curls
5. Calf Raises
6. Abs

High Intensity Interval Training (HIIT) Cardio/30min

WEDNESDAY

Abdominal Circuit 15min/ High Intensity Interval Training (HIIT) Cardio 45min

Abs 15min, 1 to 3 circuits/sets of each

Choose six abdominal exercises from the Fitness ABC Training section. Some examples have been provided below.

1. Oblique Crunches
2. Ball Crunches
3. Bicycle Crunches
4. Back Raises
5. Leg Lifts
6. Floor Crunches

Training

Example charts to keep track of your exercises for Weeks 1-4:

Upper Body	Set 1	Set 2	Set 3	Set 4	Set 5	Set 6
Chest						
Back						
Shoulders						
Biceps						
Triceps						
Abs						

Lower Body	Set 1	Set 2	Set 3	Set 4	Set 5	Set 6
Lunges						
Squats						
Leg Extension						
Leg Curls						
Calf Raises						
Abs						

Weeks 5 through 8: "Shape it up"

MONDAY/WEDNESDAY/FRIDAY

High Intensity Interval Training (HIIT) Cardio 30min/ Full Body Circuit 30min

Note: Always stretch 6-10 minutes before performing any exercise routine. We do not recommend starting any workout routine without first doing some type of warm up.

Full Body 30min, 2-4 circuits/sets of each

1. Lunges
2. Squats
3. Shoulders

4. Biceps
5. Chest
6. Back
7. Leg Extension
8. Leg Curls
9. Triceps

TUESDAY/THURSDAY

Abdominal Circuit 15min/ High Intensity Interval Training (HIIT) Cardio 45 min

Abs 15min, 1 to 3 circuits/sets of each

Choose six abdominal exercises from the Fitness ABC Training section. Some examples have been provided below.

1. Floor Crunches
2. Bench Crunches
3. Russian Twists
4. Bicycle Crunches
5. Leg Raises
6. Back Raises

Example charts to keep track of your exercises for Weeks 5-8:

Full Body	Set 1	Set 2	Set 3	Set 4
Lunges				
Squats				
Shoulders				
Biceps				
Chest				
Back				
Leg Extensions				
Leg Curls				
Triceps				

Training

Abs	Set 1	Set 2	Set 3
Floor Crunches			
Bench Crunches			
Russian Twists			
Bicycle Crunches			
Leg Raises			
Back Raises			

Weeks 9 through 12: "Dial it in"

MONDAY/WEDNESDAY/FRIDAY

Full Body Circuit 45min /Abdominal Circuit 15min

Full Body 45min, 3-6 circuits/sets of each

1. Lunges
2. Squats
3. Shoulders
4. Biceps
5. Chest
6. Back
7. Leg Extension
8. Leg Curls
9. Triceps

Abs 15min. 1 to 3 circuits/sets of each

Choose six abdominal exercises from the Fitness ABC Training section. Some examples have been provided below.

1. Floor Crunches
2. Bench Crunches
3. Russian Twists
4. Bicycle Crunches

5. Leg Raises
6. Back Raises

Example charts to keep track of your exercises for Weeks 9-12:

Full Body	Set 1	Set 2	Set 3	Set 4	Set 5	Set 6
Lunges						
Squats						
Shoulders						
Biceps						
Chest						
Back						
Leg Extensions						
Leg Curls						
Triceps						

Abs	Set 1	Set 2	Set 3
Floor Crunches			
Bench Crunches			
Russian Twists			
Bicycle Crunches			
Leg Raises			
Back Raises			

TUESDAY/THURSDAY

High Intensity Interval Training (HIIT) Cardio 1 Hour

For more tips, tools and information about The Engagement Diet, please visit our website at www.theengagementdiet.com.

Training

FITNESS ABC TRAINING

Note: The pictures provided here are visually descriptive, and so lengthy explanations about how to perform each exercise will not be provided. We recommend paying close attention to your posture at all times. Be sure to recognize whether knees should be bent or a straight leg is required. The same can be said of elbows and wrists. Always note the direction of your grip when doing the upper body circuit, and never push yourself beyond a reasonable limit when performing any of these activities.

Upper Body Circuit

CHEST

INCLINE PRESS

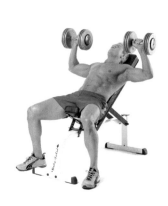
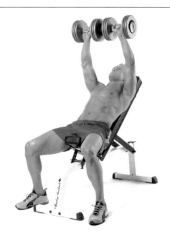

BENCH PRESS

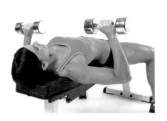
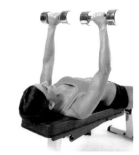

DUMBELL FLYES

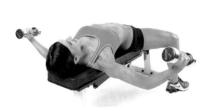
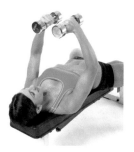

PUSH-UPS

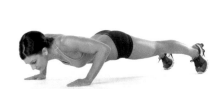
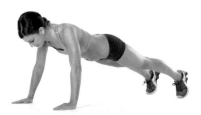

PUSH-UPS ON KNEES

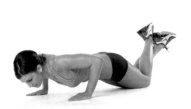
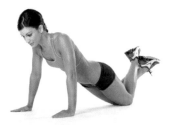

Training

DUMBBELL PUSH-UPS

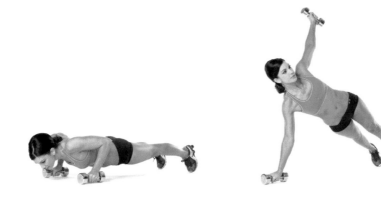

CLOSE GRIP PUSH-UP

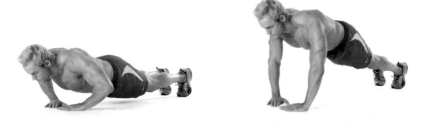

WIDE GRIP PUSH-UP

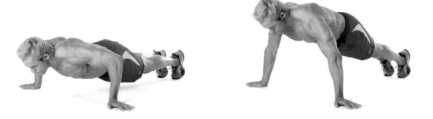

CABLE FLYES

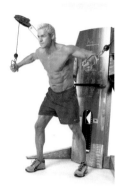
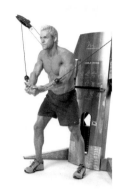

REVERSE GRIP CABLE FLYES

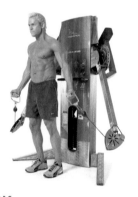
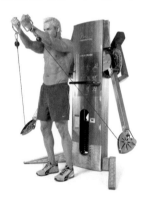

BACK

CHIN UP

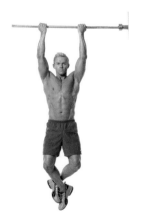
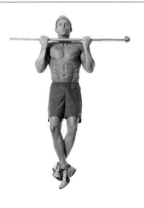

Training

153

PULL UP

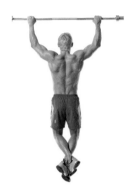
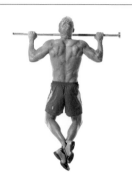

BEND-OVER ROWS WITH DUMBBELLS

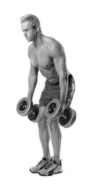
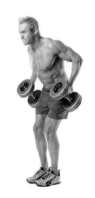

ONE ARM DUMBBELL ROW

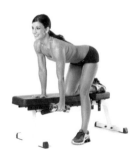
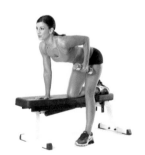

Training

LAT CABLE ROWS

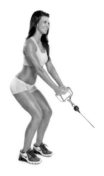 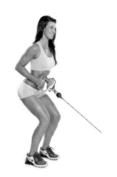

WIDE GRIP CABLE ROWS

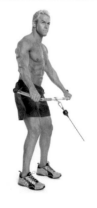 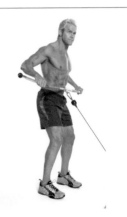

CABLE PULLOVER)

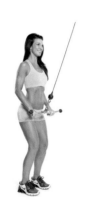 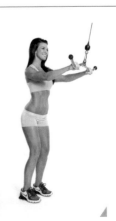

Training

LAT PULLDOWN

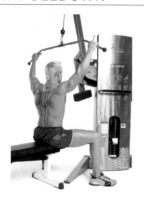 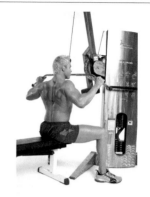

REVERSE GRIP LAT PULLDOWN

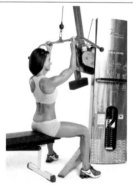 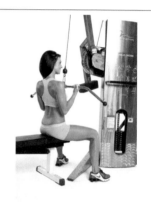

SHOULDERS

LATERAL RAISE WITH CABLES)

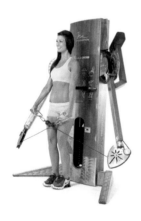 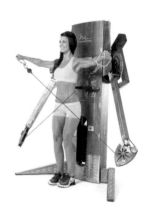

Training

REAR DELT LATERAL RAISES

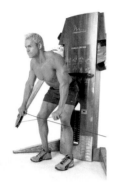 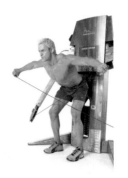

SEATED DUMBBELL PRESS

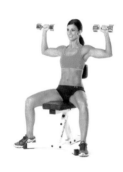 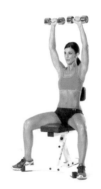

LATERAL RAISES

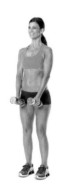 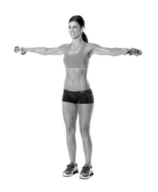

Training

BENT-OVER DUMBBELL FLYES

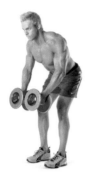 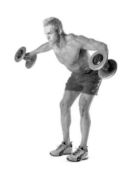

FRONT RAISES

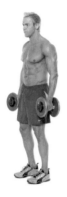 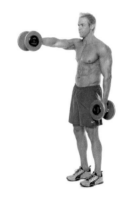

FRONT RAISES WITH PLATES

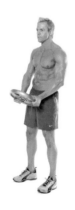 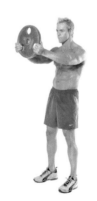

Training

FRONT RAISES WITH CABLES

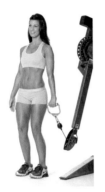 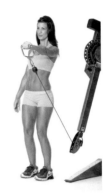

FRONT RAISES WITH REVERSE GRIP

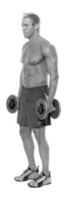 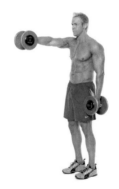

SHOULDER PRESS WITH BAND

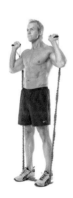 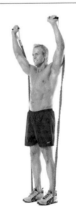

Training

LATERAL RAISE WITH BAND

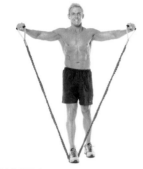 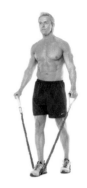

BICEPS

REVERSE BICEP CURLS

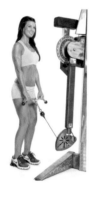 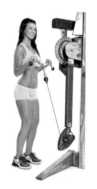

HAMMER CURLS

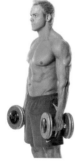 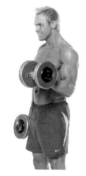

BARBELL WIDE GRIP CURLS

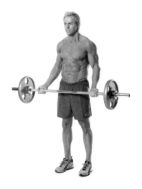 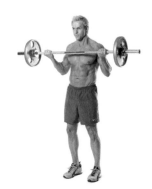

BARBELL CURLS

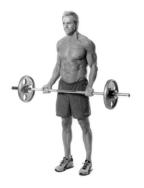 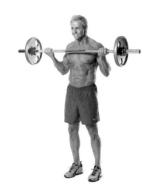

BICEP CURLS

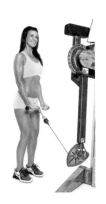 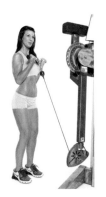

Training

BICEP CURLS

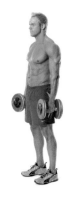
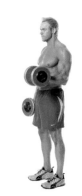

CONCENTRATION BICEP CURLS

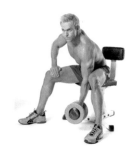
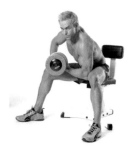

HAMMER CURL WITH CABLE

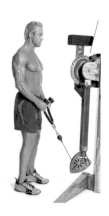
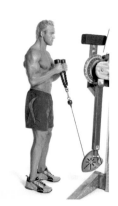

Training

BICEP CURL WITH BAND

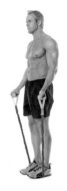 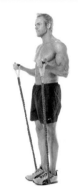

TRICEPS

TRICEP EXTENSION WITH HAMMER GRIP

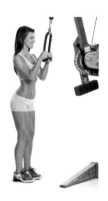 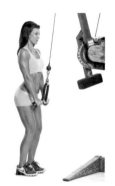

SKULL CRUSHER

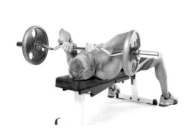 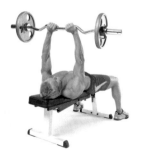

Training

TWO ARM OVERHEAD DUMBBELL EXTENSION

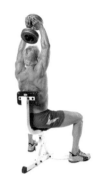
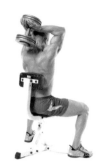

ONE ARM DUMBBELL KICK-BACK

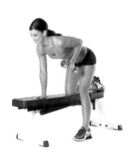
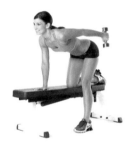

BENCH DIPS

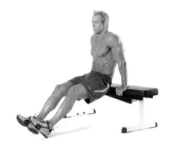
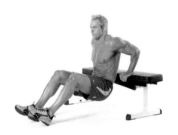

Training

TRICEP EXTENSION WITH REGULAR GRIP

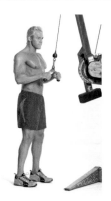 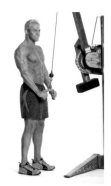

TRICEP EXTENSION WITH REVERSE GRIP

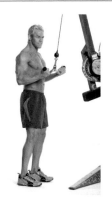 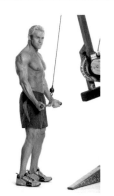

OVERHEAD TRICEP EXTENSION

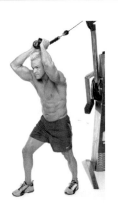 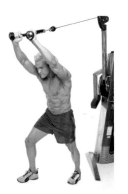

Training

Lower Body Circuit

BODY WEIGHT SQUATS

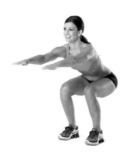

BARBELL SQUATS

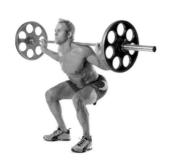
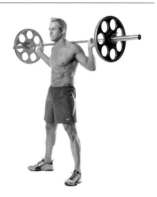

DUMBBELL SQUAT

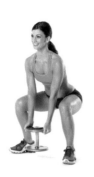
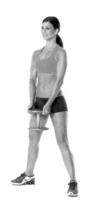

DUMBBELL LUNGES

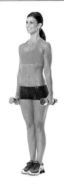
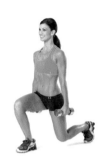

TRAVELING DUMBBELL LUNGES

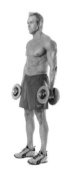
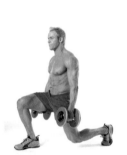
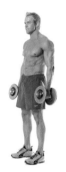
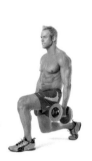

LEG EXTENSIONS

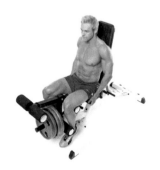
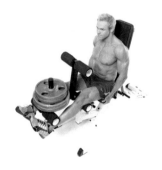

Training

LEG CURLS

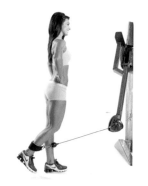 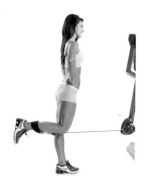

STRAIGHT LEG DEADLIFT

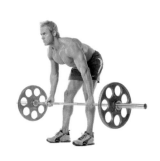 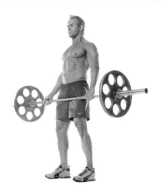

CALF RAISE

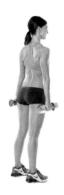 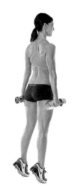

Training

CALF RAISE SEATED

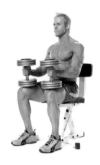 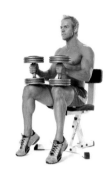

Abdominal Circuit

EXERCISE BALL CABLE AB CRUNCHES

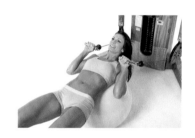 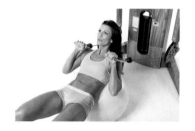

CABLE CROSS OVER

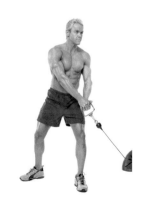 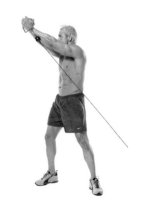

Training

CABLE SIDE CROSS OVER

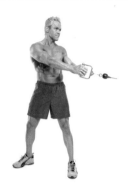 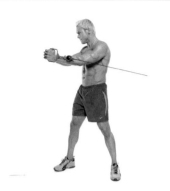

BENT KNEE LEG RAISE

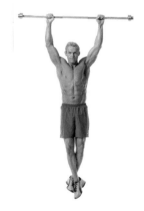 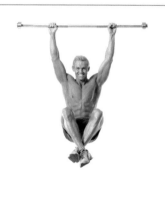

OBLIQUE LEG RAISE

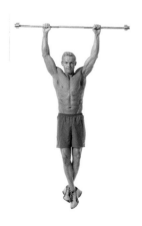 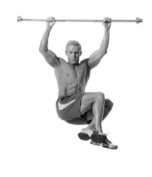

DECLINE CRUNCH WITH MEDICINE BALL

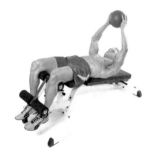 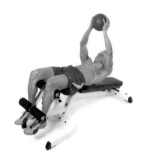

DECLINE OBLIQUE CRUNCH

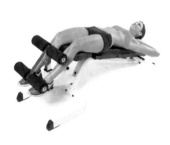 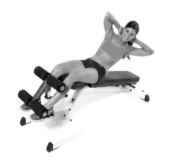

FLOOR CRUNCHES

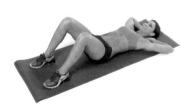 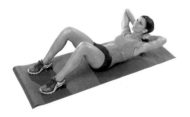

Training

LEG EXTEND CRUNCHES

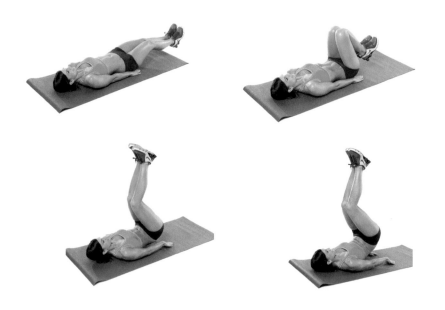

BICYCLE CRUNCHES

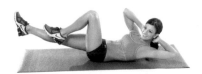

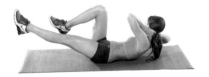

BALL-PASS CRUNCHES

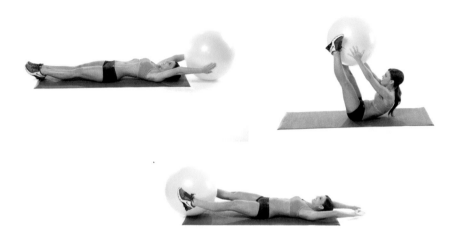

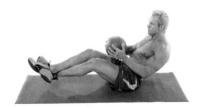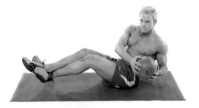

RUSSIAN TWIST WITH MEDICINE BALL

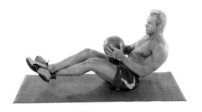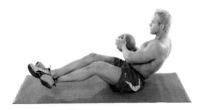

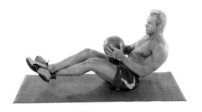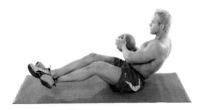

173

LOWER BACK RAISES WITH EXERCISE BALL

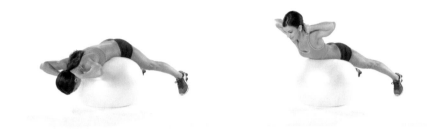

MEDICINE BALL PASS

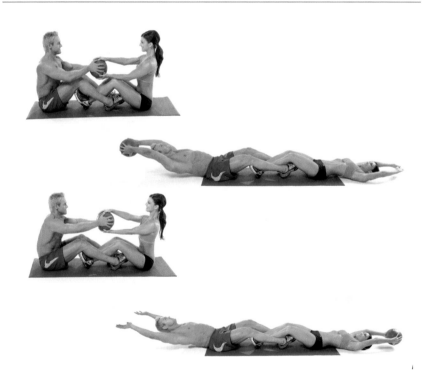

For more tips, tools and information about The Engagement Diet, please visit our website at www.theengagementdiet.com.

Training

FITNESS ABC TIPS

1. Schedule your workout. Prioritize it and protect it.

2. Pack your workout bag the night before.

3. Load your iPod with great music. Get the stuff you love. Make a playlist that keeps you going.

4. Buy good earphones. The sound will be better and it will feel better in your ears.

5. Get a water bottle that holds the right amount of water and that pours well.

6. Know your workout before you go. Print it out, write it out or simply bring this book —whatever you need to do.

7. Pick a gym you think has good energy and is located near where you will be during the time of day you will be working out.

8. Familiarize yourself with the layout of the gym and all the amenities it offers.

9. Enlist someone at the gym to show you how the machines operate. Knowing how they work and the proper form for maximum impact is essential to your success.

10. If you don't feel "on," dig deep. Persevere. Just go. Showing up is half the battle. Usually by the time you finish your warm-up, you feel better and are ready for your workout.

11. Celebrate small beginnings. Do what you can do. Do what you can do right now.

12. Train your focus on what helps you. Focus on this minute, the next ten minutes, the whole workout or the entire program. Different

Training

focal points at different times will see you through whatever you need at that moment.

13. Give yourself a break. Don't take it too seriously. This should be fun. You are doing it together.

14. Change up the cardio. Keep it fresh. Attend classes. Try new machines, like the stationary bike, recumbent bike, treadmill, and elliptical.

15. Get on a machine next to someone who can push you, or someone you can secretly compete against.

16. Make it a game. Guess your heart rate before you check it. Watch others and try to better their effort.

17. When you are "on," push it. See how long or far you can go. Surprise yourself.

18. Don't be afraid to go to the next weight. Impress yourself.

19. When you are on a set, own it. Don't worry about leaving gas in the tank.

20. If you have second thoughts once you are at the gym, put them aside. You are already there. Make the most of it.

21. Put your phone on airplane mode during your workout—no phone calls in or out. Protect this time just for you.

22. Wear clothes that you like and that make you feel good.

23. Create your gym persona. Love that person.

24. Stretch your muscles.

Training

25. Reward yourself with clothes, a fun meal or date night when you go over and above in your workout.

26. Take a large container of water to the gym. Stay hydrated. Cravings come from dehydration and tissue dehydration.

27. Stave off boredom by mixing up the cardio. Swim instead of using the machines. Take it outdoors. Sprint and walk through a scenic neighborhood.

For more tips, tools and information about The Engagement Diet, please visit our website at www.theengagementdiet.com.

Training